"I h
stres
quic
evid
at it

"I h   and can
unre

                                                        ...te Sector Division,
                                                                  Fujitsu UK

"Lea   nas never been made so easy. My
clier   ...red with this knowledge and ready for
the (...ng their thinking."

Fran Morris, Clinical Nurse Specialist, CAMHS

"Ric   ...is insights have time and time again provided a new lens
thro ...h which to look at familiar problems. He's part of our team,
a coach, and a mentor with a practical approach to our business and
personal challenges."

Rob Chapman, UK Managing Director, Unisys

"Rick provides a range of tools and techniques that ultimately allow
individuals and teams to realise their full potential."

Campbell Robertson, Managing Director,
Blenheim Consulting Ltd

"The methodolo   nitive-
behavioural and   n pick
up and follow in

                                                                 Nurse,
                                                                 liance

About the author

Dr Rick Norris is a chartered psychologist, writer, and lecturer, and works as an executive coach with a range of corporations from Fujitsu and Nokia-Siemens to Thomas Cook Airlines. He is a director of Mind Health Development Ltd, through which he runs training workshops for mental health practitioners. He also continues to work as a clinical psychologist in private practice offering support to sufferers of stress, anxiety, and depression using cognitive-behavioural techniques.

THINK YOURSELF HAPPY

The simple 6-step programme to
change your life from within

RICK NORRIS

ONEWORLD
OXFORD

A Oneworld Book
Published by Oneworld Publications 2011
Copyright © Rick Norris 2010

ISBN 978–1–85168–777–0

Typeset by Glyph International, Bangalore
Cover design by vaguelymemorable.com
Printed and bound in Great Britain by Page Bros

Oneworld Publications
185 Banbury Road, Oxford, OX2 7AR, England

Learn more about Oneworld. Join our mailing list
to find out about our latest titles and special offers at:
www.oneworld-publications.com

To all the people I have had the privilege of helping over the years. You have all been brave enough to face your demons and come through stronger than you were before. I salute you.

CONTENTS

Introduction

If you're unhappy with your life, this book will be able to help. *Think Yourself Happy* provides simple explanations for understanding the causes of stress, anxiety and depression and lots of practical exercises, tips and techniques to overcome these problems. When you've learned the six steps to change your life from within, you'll become more fulfilled in every aspect of your life.

At the beginning of my favourite film, *Butch Cassidy and the Sundance Kid*, we see the words: 'Most of what follows is true'. It's the same with this book. I've spent many years as a psychologist counselling numerous people suffering from various forms of stress, anxiety and depression. Some of their stories are recorded here; although the stories are true, I've changed the details to protect their identities. Every story I've used is based on real-life experience; hopefully this will make them easier to understand and identify with.

How to use this book

This isn't a theoretical textbook; it's a practical tool to help you think about your life. Be bold: **don't be afraid of writing in the book**. Underline the bits you identify with, make notes on subjects you want to reflect on later, capture your thoughts as you go along and use the summaries at the end of each step – this will help improve your understanding and memory. Make the effort to complete the exercises and refer back to them so you can reflect on the progress you're making. This will make the book much more personal and the answers might encourage you to think realistically about yourself. You might come to some unexpected conclusions.

My colleague Glyn and I have successfully used these steps with thousands of clients over the years. There are three reasons why they are so effective. First, the simple explanations give people the clarity they need to understand what's going on in their minds. Second, the practical exercises and techniques are easy to complete. Last, and most important, my clients regularly practise the techniques. If you follow these guidelines, they'll work for you too. However, please remember this book isn't a magic potion. Be patient: if you've been unhappy for months or even years, you'll need to practise the steps for a little while before you start to gain the benefits but eventually you will learn all the steps to think yourself happy!

Feeling stressed, anxious or depressed can often be a very lonely experience. Yet the reality, as we shall see in Step 1, is that many people suffer from psychological health problems.

Research suggests that it can help to share our experiences with others,[1] so if you have specific questions for Glyn or me, contact us via the website www.mindhealthdevelopment.co.uk. We promise to respond to all your comments.

Thank you
Rick

STEP 1   ❦

Recognise that you are not alone

At the start of an episode of the television series *Cheers*, the character Norm walks into the bar. Woody the barman calls out 'Hi, Norm, how's life?' To which Norm replies 'Not for the fainthearted.' Norm is right. Life can be very daunting at times; the twenty-first century world is a very complex and potentially stressful place for everyone.

Into every life a little rain must fall

If you're reading this book the chances are that you're not as happy with your life as you'd like to be. You're not alone; whether you're rich or poor, black or white, gay or straight – into every life a little rain must fall. It's this rain that makes us feel stressed, anxious or depressed.

All my clients have their fair share of troubles but when they first come to see me I like to find out about them as people before I ask them about their difficulties. Finding out about each person is important; everyone is individual, with their own personality, their own experiences, their own work circumstances, their own dreams and their own troubles.

Who are you? What words best describe you?

- ....
- ....
- ....
- ....

What kind of work do you do?

- ....
- ....
- ....
- ....

What are the most important relationships in your life?

- ....
- ....
- ....
- ....

What's your social life like?

- ....
- ....
- ....
- ....

What is your deepest dream?

- ....
- ....
- ....
- ....

What gets in the way of your happiness?

- ....
- ....
- ....
- ....

Hopefully it didn't take you more than a few minutes to jot down some information about yourself. Throughout this book, you'll have the opportunity to learn some valuable steps that will help you understand yourself better. Armed with that knowledge, you'll be better equipped to look more objectively at your life and I'll give you the skills to help you deal with your troubles and make your dreams and goals a reality.

Almost everyone has a few troubles. Although the numbers vary, statistics suggest that stress, anxiety and depression are very common. One in six people will suffer from significant mental health problems during their lives[2] and one in four will suffer some form of psychological ill-health.[3] It's probably safe to say that almost everyone will experience some form of stress, anxiety or depression at some point in their lives. You're not alone: it's a modern-day plague.

What do we mean by *stress, anxiety* and *depression*?

Believe it or not, there are about three hundred different types of anxiety and mood disorders! The list includes post-traumatic stress, obsessive-compulsive disorder, phobias, panic attacks, depression, bipolar disorder (manic depression) and major depression.[4] These terms can be quite confusing, so let's try to simplify them.

Stress is the feeling we experience when we are faced with challenges. Minor stressful challenges could include events such as making a business presentation or going on a first date.

Think of a recent occasion when you felt stressed: what caused it?

- ....
- ....
- ....
- ....

What thoughts were going through your head?

- ....
- ....
- ....
- ....

What physical reactions did you experience?

- ....
- ....
- ....
- ....

The stress of a minor challenge is short-lived. Once the event is over, the stress gradually disappears; the normal reaction to a minor challenge. However, major challenges can produce stress levels that may be more difficult to deal with successfully. Major challenges often come in the form of life events, such as dealing with the death of a close relative, becoming unemployed, a relationship breaking up or experiencing serious illness/injury. Some life events may be broadly positive but at the same time stressful: we may look forward to the birth of a child or moving house but these events can also bring their fair share of stress.

Think of a recent life event you've experienced. How did it make you feel?

- ....
- ....
- ....
- ....

How long did it last and how did it continue to affect you?

- ....
- ....
- ....
- ....

Most of the time, we cope with stress reasonably well but at certain times we can become overloaded, either with multiple life events or a single life event which seems to drag on forever. Later, we'll look at life events in more detail to understand why this happens.

Anxiety is a feeling of apprehension or fear. It can result from the stress we experience from either a minor or major challenge. In many ways mild anxiety is a normal and healthy response to a challenge because it helps us prepare to meet it. However anxiety disorders produce very strong or longer-lasting feelings which cause more severe reactions.

Think of a time when you felt really fearful or apprehensive. Was it something specific that caused quite strong feelings of fear or was it a more generalised nagging anxiety?

- ....
- ....
- ....
- ....

What physical reactions did you experience?

- ....
- ....
- ....
- ....

Anxiety disorders can be acute or chronic. Acute anxiety is often sparked by a particular trigger that causes quite intense symp-toms such as panic attacks. Although it seems to go on forever, normally, the effects of acute anxiety don't last very long. The Olympic gold medal-winning cyclist, Chris Hoy, is a good example of a person who suffered from acute anxiety. Early in his career, Chris was plagued with performance anxiety; before a big race, he would begin to panic, worrying whether he was good enough or whether he would be able to live up to everyone's expectations. His palms would sweat, his legs would turn to jelly and he would feel a huge sense of dread. However, using techniques similar to those in this book, Chris was able to overcome this acute anxiety.

People who suffer from chronic anxiety experience long-term feelings of dread and apprehension. Their reactions are less intense than those of people who suffer from acute anxiety but the effects last much longer. Chronic anxiety often doesn't have a specific trigger; it can be a general feeling, which used to be described as 'free-floating' anxiety. One client I worked with, Indira, exhibited symptoms of free-floating anxiety. Nothing specific was directly causing her anxiety; she just worried about lots of situations in her work, home and personal life.

Depression is a state of mind rather than a specific feeling. A depressive state of mind usually results in a serious, long-term, lowering of enjoyment of life and/or an inability to visualise a happy future. People who suffer from severe depression take no pleasure from life and frequently lose all hope.

Have you ever felt depressed? Do you know how the depression started?

- ....

How long did it last?

- ....

How did it affect other areas of your life?

- ....

- ....
- ....
- ....

Depression can develop over time or it can be brought on by major life events. Eamon was a forty-year-old client whose wife had died in a car accident. He was left to care for their three children as well as working full time. Unsurprisingly, poor Eamon became depressed and found it very hard to find any enjoyment in life while he attempted to come to terms with this painful and difficult situation.

Two factors combine to produce a depressed state of mind. First, depressed people play negative thoughts over and over again (negative introspection). Second, they stop doing things, especially the things they used to enjoy. Someone diagnosed with severe depression will often spend hours lying in bed or sitting at home constantly thinking negative thoughts.

Increased levels of anxiety can cause both depression and anxiety disorders. However, we can experience anxiety disorders without going on to experience depression. Equally, we can experience depression without having an anxiety disorder. If we're really unlucky, we can experience both anxiety disorders and depression.

How the brain reacts to stressful challenges

As you completed the previous exercises about how you felt when you were stressed, anxious or depressed, no doubt you'll have written down some of your physical and psychological reactions.

My colleague Glyn uses a character he calls 'cave man Dave' to explain how the brain reacts to a stressful challenge. If cave man Dave were out hunting for food and he came across a dangerous wild animal, his brain would switch on his sympathetic nervous system (SNS), flooding Dave's body with the hormone adrenaline. The body's response to adrenaline – traditionally known as the 'fight or flight' response – would help Dave either to fight or run away from the wild animal. Once Dave had either got away safely or killed the beast, his brain would switch off his SNS and his adrenaline levels would subside.

Some stress and anxiety is a perfectly normal reaction to the challenges we face every day. As we can see from cave man Dave, it helps us to deal with challenges effectively. However, because many of our modern-day challenges are complicated psychological challenges, which can worry us for long periods of time (rather than simple and immediate physical challenges such as being chased by wild animals), it's not so easy to switch the SNS off. Earlier, when you completed the exercise on anxiety, I asked you to think about a time when you were fearful or apprehensive. As you were recalling this memory, your SNS may have started producing adrenaline. The more vivid the memory then the more adrenaline you would have produced.

Think of a time when you felt really relaxed and happy – perhaps a memory of a walk in the country or spending time with friends or family. Take three or four minutes to recall what you could see, hear, smell, touch or taste (it may help to close your eyes)

- ....
- ....
- ....
- ....

Describe your mood now. How do you feel?

- ....
- ....
- ....
- ....

When we feel relaxed and positive, or we take part in enjoyable activities, the parasympathetic nervous system (PNS) releases neurotransmitters, such as serotonin and norepinephrine, which results in a positive mood. In short, the PNS gives us the 'feel-good factor'.

The SNS and PNS can't both be switched on together: we can't feel stressed and relaxed at the same time! If we feel constantly challenged, stressed and anxious, the SNS will be switched on and the PNS switched off. With the switch for the SNS jammed on, the body is continuously flooded with adrenaline. This means that the PNS is locked off, reducing the amount of neurotransmitters being produced.

If we experience lots of stress, and the SNS is constantly switched on, we can eventually suffer from anxiety disorders or depression, with both psychological and physiological effects. Psychological effects include a range of problems such as irrational worries and fears, inability to concentrate, making errors even on simple tasks, experiencing strong negative emotions

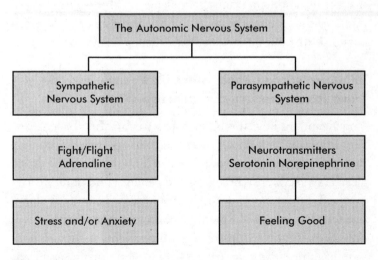

Figure 1

such as anger or sadness in response to minor incidents, numbness to any feeling at all and feeling suicidal. The physiological symptoms are just as varied: sleeplessness, loss of appetite, skin disorders, depletion of the immune system (leading to increased risk of infections) and high blood pressure. Even heart disease and cancer are implicated as symptoms of psychological illness.

It's not surprising that if we feel stressed, anxious or depressed, we may decide to visit the doctor. Every year, millions of people visit their GP for psychological problems – further evidence that you're not alone. Doctors often prescribe antidepressants to try to help but it's important to understand that antidepressants are only designed to deal with the chemical imbalance in the brain, not the negative thinking patterns at the root of the problem. While antidepressants may make people feel better in the short term, they're not a long-term solution and aren't licensed for extended use. The most effective long-term solution for psychological problems is to learn the steps in this book, to help you to think more positively. More information on antidepressants is available on the website www.mindhealthdevelopment.co.uk but this should not replace discussion with your GP or a qualified mental health practitioner.

Why are some people more likely to suffer from stress, anxiety and depression?

Understanding how the brain reacts to stressful challenges is very important but it's a mistake to think of anxiety disorders or depression just as chemical imbalances.[5] Although imbalance clearly is a factor, psychological and genetic conditions are also involved. Some mood disorders are inherited but even someone who has inherited a predisposition to a mood disorder will only be susceptible to psychological problems if they suffer a significant negative experience.[6] People who suffer a significant negative experience in early life seem to be more prone to psychological problems later on in life.

Think about your childhood and teenage years. What were the positive things you experienced when you were growing up?

- ....
- ....
- ....
- ....

What challenges or difficulties did you face in your early years?

- ....
- ....
- ....
- ....

Threat sensitivity

My experience as a psychologist suggests that many of (though by no means all) the people I've counselled had difficulties in their early life. As a result, they became 'threat sensitive' quite early in their childhood or adolescence. Ordinarily, we don't experience serious life events in childhood or, if we do, hopefully we'll remain relatively protected from them by our parents. However sometimes children suffer deeply from negative experiences and are often unable to verbalise them, which can lead to threat sensitivity. From an early age, threat sensitive people are more likely to notice potentially negative aspects of life. Although we all experience life events (into every life a little rain must fall!), threat sensitive people are affected more deeply and find it harder to cope with them. They are also more susceptible to stress, anxiety and depression.

I've noticed that people who suffer from threat sensitivity seem to have been exposed to at least one of three early life experiences. The first is the effect of threat sensitive parents, whether through nature or nurture. Threat sensitive parents can pass this predisposition on to their children genetically (nature), or influence their children by repeatedly telling them to be careful or warning them of the dangers of doing or not doing certain things (nurture). The second type of experience is exposure to a life event that caused general anxiety for a time: a nasty divorce, the death or serious illness of a parent or moving house or school several times.

The third type of early life experience is when something very traumatic happens in childhood or adolescence, for example mental, physical or sexual abuse. Traumas such as these are quite different from life events. Life events, although often sad and stressful, are fairly normal, whereas trauma results from unusual, if not abnormal, experiences. It's not difficult to see why threat sensitivity results from traumatic experiences.

If one of these three experiences featured in your answers to the questions on your childhood and teenage years you may, through no fault of your own, be more susceptible to psychological ill-health. In Step 3, we'll look in more detail at what makes people more susceptible to psychological ill-health.

A twenty-first century plague?

While threat sensitive people are more prone to psychological distress, this doesn't explain why the problem is so widespread. To understand, we need to look at the environmental factors that have contributed to making psychological ill-health a twenty-first century plague.

Stress and work

As recently as the 1950s, people had a much simpler relationship with the world of work. It was fairly typical for a person to stay with the same employer for their whole working life; there were fewer choices of job and primarily people worked to have enough money to live. In the twenty-first century, it's very different. It was recently calculated that the average American, with two years of college education, will change jobs eleven times before retirement.[7] Although the reasons for changing job are many – promotion, dissatisfaction, redundancy or dismissal – generally, the twenty-first century workplace is much less stable than its 1950s counterpart.

What's your current job?

- ....
- ....
- ....
- ....

How long have you been in your current job? How long were you in your previous job?

- ....
- ....
- ....
- ....

What do you like about your job?

- ....
- ....
- ....
- ....

What do you dislike about your job?

- ....
- ....
- ....
- ....

How much sickness absence have you had in the last twelve months?

- ....
- ....
- ....
- ....

In the twenty-first century, work seems to be one of the main sources of stress, anxiety and depression. Despite the evidence that modern workplaces are safer than ever and we are, in relative terms, much better paid than our parents or grandparents, we continue to see worrying trends in sickness absence from work. A Japanese study suggested that a hugely disproportionate percentage of heart attacks are suffered on Monday mornings, when people are getting ready to start their working week.[8] The stress some people experience at the thought of beginning another working week can lead to significant surges in blood pressure, which can cause heart attacks.

If you noted that you've had time off work because you were stressed, it's another example of why you're not alone. According to a recent report, mental ill health is the second-largest cause of sickness absence in UK organisations.[9] Interestingly, one survey pointed the finger at work itself as a significant source of stress, suggesting that 14% of the working population experienced work-related stress at a level that made them ill.[10]

Even if we really enjoy our work, it can still be difficult to get the right balance between our work and personal lives. In the 1950s, it was easier; in the twenty-first century it has become much more difficult to know where the boundaries lie. One of the main causes of the blurring of our work/life boundaries is technology. We are far more accessible than we used to be: mobile phones mean it's easy for work colleagues to call us about a problem regardless of where we are; portable computers and other devices with fast connections to the Internet mean we can take work with us whenever and wherever we want. I've counselled dozens of people who've told me that the only way they can keep up with the pressure of work is to take it home. However, while it's easy to put the blame for our difficulty in achieving a work/life balance on our employer's expectations, lots of us want to work from home.[11]

I once worked with an IT director, Guy, who lived and worked just outside London. He proposed to his boss that he should spend one week a month working from his holiday home in Spain. His mobile phone worked in Spain, he had a fast Internet connection there, he could join in conference calls at any time and if he were required to return to the UK quickly, there were several daily flights from a number of nearby airports. Unfortunately, Guy's boss turned down the proposal, because he couldn't see past the fact that if Guy were in his holiday home, then he must be on holiday, not at work. This example highlights just how complex the balance between work and life can be but if we don't get it right, it's easy to suffer from stress, anxiety or depression.

Changes in family life and the community

Sometimes it's difficult to know whether work stress negatively affects our personal life, whether the stress in our personal lives negatively affects our work – or both. What does seem to be clear is that the complexity of life in the twenty-first century has significantly affected our lives.

Where do you live?
- ....
- ....
- ....
- ....

With whom do you live?

- ....
- ....
- ....
- ....

How long have you lived there?

- ....
- ....
- ....
- ....

How well do you know your neighbours?

- ....
- ....
- ....
- ....

How friendly are you with the people in your neighbourhood?

- ....
- ....
- ....
- ....

Family life and communities have changed radically since the 1970s. We live in a much more geographically mobile society. Social commentators suggest that 1970s neighbourhoods with even the loosest community ties would be regarded as strong communities by twenty-first century standards. In the 1950s, family members – grandparents, aunts, uncles and cousins – often lived locally, frequently in the same street, sometimes in the same house; today, families are dispersed across countries or even continents. Neighbours often worked at the same company or factory; today, people commute from dormitory towns to hundreds of different workplaces in large cities. Streets of back-to-back terraced housing meant that neighbours were physically close, which encouraged community spirit; today, many communities were destroyed as these houses were pulled down.

Perhaps one of the most significant factors in the rise in mental health problems is the increase in the breakdown of relationships. Separation and divorce are more common now than they've ever been. In the UK in 1961, there were just over 27,000 divorces; in 2008, there were 136,000. Not only is the divorce rate much higher but the number of marriages has steadily declined, from a peak of more than 480,000 in 1972 to 270,000 in 2008. In the same period, the population increased from 56 million to 62 million, so it's pretty clear that relationships are a lot less stable in the twenty-first century.[12]

Your answers to the exercise on 'where do you live' may reflect these statistics. The chances are your answers will be very different to those your grandparents or even your parents would have given at your age.

Think about the house, the family and the neighbourhood you grew up in as a child. How was it different to where you live now?

- ....
- ....
- ....
- ....

Higher expectations

Psychological health problems appear to be a global problem. More than 25% of the population of both developed and developing countries is likely to suffer from some type of mental health problem.[13] However, it seems that in the West, depression in particular is linked to higher – and often unrealistic – expectations. We want it all and we want it now!

In the twenty-first century, in developed countries, most of our basic needs are met with relative ease. Even if we aren't able to work, welfare and social security mean that very few people die of starvation or exposure to the elements. Consequently our expectations are much higher. We want a great relationship with an attractive and interesting partner, well-behaved and lovely children, a spacious house, a new car, several foreign holidays a year, a well-paid job and good friends to socialise with. Beyond the tangible rewards, we want to be appreciated, respected and cared for, to be consulted and involved in the decisions affecting our lives, to have the opportunity to use and develop our talents and to feel that we add value and make a difference. Unfortunately we don't have a god-given right to any of them. And when these – sometimes unrealistic – expectations are not met, we are likely to suffer from anxiety and depression. Having more realistic expectations of life sets us up for success; we're more likely to achieve them and therefore our levels of satisfaction with life are likely to be much higher.

Are all your expectations realistic? Which of your expectations may be unrealistic?

- ....
- ....
- ....
- ....

Summary of Step 1

If you're suffering from stress, anxiety or depression, you are not alone – psychological ill-health is very common. We live in a complex, twenty-first century world in which, despite the fact that there are about three hundred types of mental disorder, our brains still react to challenges in the same way as cave man Dave's. Although we all share the same structures in the sympathetic and parasympathetic nervous systems, some people are more threat sensitive than others and therefore more likely to develop psychological health problems. Certain genetic and psychological factors explain why some of us are more threat sensitive than others but environmental factors also explain why our twenty-first century world is potentially a more threat sensitive place in which to live.

Into every life a little rain must fall

If you're not as happy with your life as you'd like to be, you're not alone. Into every life a little rain must fall and it's the rain that makes us feel stressed, anxious or depressed. Stress is the feeling we experience when faced with challenges. Anxiety is a feeling of apprehension and fear, which can result from the stress of a challenge. Mild anxiety is quite normal, unlike anxiety disorders. Depression is a state of mind resulting in serious, long-term lowering of enjoyment of life or the inability to visualise a happy future.

How the brain reacts to stressful challenges

The autonomic nervous system has two parts: the sympathetic nervous system (SNS) and the parasympathetic nervous system (PNS). If the SNS is jammed on and the PNS is locked off, this causes a chemical imbalance.

Why are some people more likely to suffer from stress, anxiety and depression?

Threat sensitivity results from exposure to at least one of three experiences in early life: the effect of threat sensitive parents, a life event or a trauma.

A twenty-first century plague?

Stress and work: the difficulty in achieving a healthy work/ life balance has contributed to the increase in psychological health problems. Changes in family life and the community have resulted in much less support for people suffering from psychological health problems. Higher expectations: unrealistic expectations set us up for failure, which can contribute to feelings of stress, anxiety and depression.

In the next step we'll look at what goes on in our minds as we succumb to the stresses of the twenty-first century world.

S T E P 2 ✀

Understand how your negative mind works

T hreat sensitivity is linked to stress, anxiety and depression but how does our negative mind work?

The mind: the DVD library and the DVD player

The mind operates at both subconscious and conscious levels. The subconscious mind is like a library full of DVDs, on which our memories and thoughts are recorded and then stored on the shelves. The conscious mind is the DVD player on which we replay those thoughts and memories. Most psychologists believe in the theory of *permanent memory*, that everything we experience is stored away in the mind's subconscious library. However, our recall system isn't very good and we often struggle to recall memories at will.

What you were doing fifteen years ago? Where were you living?

- ....
- ....
- ....
- ....

What did your house look like?

- ....
- ....
- ....
- ....

What job were you doing?

- ....
- ....
- ....
- ....

Who was your boss/your best work mate?

- ....
- ....
- ....
- ....

What car did you drive?

- ....
- ....
- ....
- ....

To recall what you were doing fifteen years ago you trawled the library to find the DVDs recorded at that time of your life. You probably haven't replayed some of those memories for a very long time; they may not be particularly relevant to your life now. The more relevant something is, the more likely we are to replay DVDs relating to it. However, if you were listening to the radio and heard a popular song from fifteen years ago, you might instantly recall memories from that time. The DVDs are stacked on the shelves of our mental library but sometimes we need a trigger, either conscious or subconscious, to start replaying a particular memory. Popular songs are often such triggers.

Some of the DVDs in the library are of positive memories, some are of negative memories and many seem to be neutral. Faced with difficult and upsetting problems, we tend to replay negative memories that are *relevant* to our difficulties. If the stressful situation persists, after a while we can find it increasingly difficult to replay positive DVDs. Constantly replaying negative memories can cause the chemical imbalances I talked about in Step 1. For example, if you'd just been made redundant from your job, it would be quite understandable if your thoughts were mainly negative for a while. The negative thoughts might include financial worries, fear of not getting another job, the pressure on your family or your lack of self-esteem through not having a job.

Think about something that's troubling you at the moment: what DVDs come into your mind?

- ....
- ....
- ....
- ....

How does it make you feel when you play these negative DVDs?

- ....
- ....
- ....
- ....

Negative DVDs can soon become frequent, invasive thoughts that are difficult to stop. The thoughts are set off by triggers, which can be either conscious or subconscious. Conscious triggers are obvious: for example, when an unemployed person hears the word 'job' they are reminded they don't have one. However, sometimes we start to replay a negative memory but without knowing why; the trigger is subconscious.

Maureen's experience is an example of a subconscious trigger causing negative DVDs to start replaying. Maureen had had a very stressful time in her previous job in the busy accident and emergency department of a large hospital. Eventually, she decided to leave and moved to a job in the local authority's housing services. However, on her first day, she experienced negative memories of her old job spinning around her head. This seemed to happen every morning but the thoughts became less invasive as the day went on. After a while, Maureen identified the subconscious trigger for the negative memories: the cleaners at the local authority used the same brand of floor polish as those at the hospital. The smell of the freshly cleaned floor subconsciously evoked memories of the hospital.

There's no such thing as a random thought!

Quickly think of something that appears to be really random.

- ....
- ....

- ....
- ....

Ask yourself how this thought came into your head; to what was it related?

- ....
- ....
- ....
- ....

Was it related to a thought you had earlier in the day?

- ....
- ....
- ....
- ....

Was it related to something in your immediate physical environment, something you could see, hear or smell?

- ....
- ....
- ....
- ....

Most DVDs start to play because they're prompted by other memories or by something we sense, something we see, hear, feel, taste or, as in Maureen's case, smell. But often, we're not *consciously* aware of the prompts.

In whatever way the memories are triggered, sometimes we find it hard to press the player's stop button and eject the negative DVD. The continuous replaying of these invasive memories starts negative thinking patterns that eventually lead to negative 'memories' being created about the future. In short, if we constantly worry about past negative events we're more likely to worry about the future. When I use the word 'memory', it can relate to both past events and possible future outcomes.

The brain's filter

Between the subconscious mind and the conscious mind lies a cluster of brain cells – the reticular activating system (RAS) – that 'filters' relevant memories from the subconscious mind's library into the conscious mind's DVD player.

As quickly as you can, count up how many Ds there are in Figure 2.

D	G	O	D	O	C	G	D	O	G
O	C	D	C	O	G	G	O	G	C
D	C	D	O	O	C	Q	G	G	D
O	C	G	D	O	O	O	G	G	D
O	Q	O	G	D	C	G	G	D	C
G	O	G	G	O	C	D	C	O	O

Figure 2

There were 12 Ds. Give yourself a pat on the back if you got it right.

Without looking at the grid again (no cheating!) can you remember how many different letters there were?

• ....

Can you remember which letter occurred the fewest times?

* ....

Roughly how many times did that letter appear?

* ....

Go back to the grid and check your answers.

The RAS is an extremely powerful mechanism. As you quickly scanned the grid, your eyes saw every single letter and your brain recorded them in your subconscious mind. However, the only letters we can be certain got through the RAS filter into your conscious mind were the Ds. By asking you to count them, I primed your filter to allow the Ds into your conscious mind. Your answers to the other questions will depend on what got through your filter. You *saw* all the other letters but you may not have *noticed* them. If you're trying to sell your house you notice every 'sold' sign. If you're trying to get pregnant, you notice every mum with a young baby. If you're saving hard to buy a new red sports car, you notice every red sports car on the road.

The filter also seems to operate through all our senses, not just sight. Sitting with a friend in a busy café, I was describing to her how the RAS filter works and she was listening intently. Over her shoulder, I could see a mother and baby at the next table. A few moments earlier, the baby had been crying and the mother had rocked it back to sleep. I asked my friend whether she'd heard the sound of a baby crying several seconds before. My friend paused for a moment and said, 'Yes, but I hadn't noticed until you mentioned it.' The sound had remained in her subconscious, only passing through the filter when I drew her attention to it. She *heard* the sound but she didn't *notice* it. The filter can also work with our sense of touch: a skilful pickpocket can steal a victim's watch without them noticing. The pick-pocket distracts the victim's conscious mind, by drawing their attention to something else, so that the feeling of having the watch removed remains in the victim's subconscious and doesn't make it through the filter to the conscious mind. They *feel* the watch being removed but they don't *notice* it.

The filter operates in much the same way for people experiencing stress, anxiety disorders or depression. Over time, their filter is programmed to notice only those things related to their troubles. They may see, hear or feel positive things in their lives but they remain unnoticed and don't get through the filter.

The RAS filter has evolved as a protective mechanism that helps identify threats but if it becomes unbalanced, it can cause problems. When it's working well, the filter protects us by allowing through a healthy balance of negative, neutral and positive memories. Mild stress and anxiety is a perfectly normal, healthy reaction to a threat. However, if the filter is working deficiently, it goes into threat identification overdrive and only allows through negative DVDs of past failures or potential threats and dangers. This causes undue anxiety to creep into a situation, increases anxiety levels, causes self-doubt and begins to destroy our confidence.

Conscious Mind
(the DVD player)
plays only negative DVDs
related to the problems

The Filter blocks positive
and neutral DVDs

Subconscious Mind
(the DVD library)
stores negative, positive,
and neutral DVDs

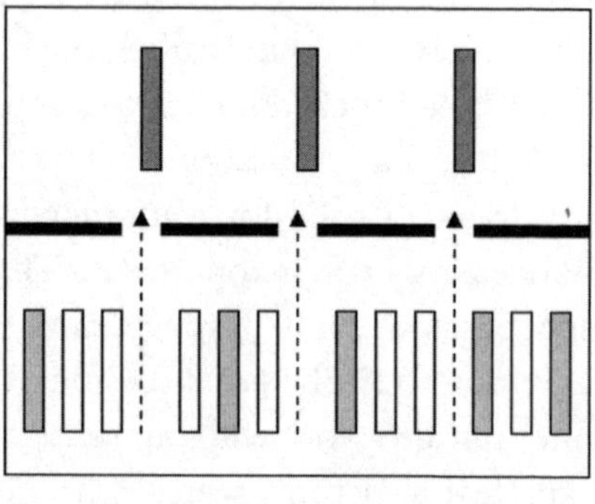

Figure 3

After his divorce, a friend of mine, Bill, spent some time looking for a new house. He ended up buying a house in a village next to the one where his ex-wife, Diane, lived. The house had been owned by Diane's Aunt Helen, a very keen gardener, who had died a couple of years earlier. In the middle of the back lawn, Helen had created a very attractive feature from a beautiful wrought-iron water pump and a large stone trough but the garden had become very overgrown since her death. Bill decided to clear all the shrubs and trees, take up the lawn and replace it with stone chippings, earthenware pots and a variety of plants; fortunately, Bill's new girlfriend, Emma, offered to help him. Bill mentioned to Emma that he intended to give the trough and water pump to Diane, as a reminder of her Aunt Helen. Emma was surprised, remarking how expensive these features would be to replace. Bill felt it would be a kind gesture to give them to Diane, as she had been very fond of her Aunt Helen.

Emma became very quiet; Bill sensed she was anxious about the apparently strong connection to his ex-wife that the gift of the pump and trough seemed to symbolise. Bill tried to convince her that she was reading too much into the gesture and eventually, Emma seemed reassured. Later that day, Bill and Emma decided to go for a walk around the village in the late evening sunshine, something they'd done quite often. After their walk, they stopped off in one of the village pubs. As they were enjoying their drinks, Emma suddenly said to Bill, 'Do you know how many black iron water pumps there are in this village?' Laughing, she recounted the location of seven or eight water pumps dotted in various gardens about the village. Despite the fact she had often walked round the village, Emma had never noticed the water pumps. She'd seen them but they remained in her subconscious mind, unnoticed. However, because Helen's pump represented something negative that troubled her, Emma's filter was activated to consciously notice all the pumps in the village.

The subconscious mind is very powerful and can operate in an almost magical way, particularly when we're facing an immediate danger. When the danger is potentially life-threatening and we need a quick reaction, we can respond to something of which we are only subconsciously aware.

In the 1950s, the Argentinian driver Juan Fangio dominated the sport of motor racing, several times becoming world champion. During one race, at a circuit with a blind left-hand bend at one point on the race track, something strange happened. A few laps into the race, Fangio approached the bend and began to brake gently, so he could negotiate the bend at the correct speed. However, he found himself unable to take his foot off the brake pedal. For some reason, he braked far harder and for much longer than normal for this type of bend. As he rounded the bend, he saw there had been a crash involving several other cars. Had Fangio not slowed down considerably, he would have smashed straight into the wrecked cars. However, he was able to negotiate his way safely around the crash and went on to win the race. Commentators marvelled at Fangio's uncanny ability to anticipate an accident that he couldn't have seen. Fangio himself was worried about what had happened, because he couldn't understand what had made him brake so much harder than normal. He was anxious that if he found himself in a similar situation, he might not be able to 'sense' his way out of danger a second time.

Fangio's subconscious mind had noticed something that caused him to brake uncharacteristically hard. A few months later, he woke up with the answer; driving along the straight approaching the left-hand bend, the main grandstand with all the spectators had been on his right. Fangio was the world champion; he was used to seeing the spectators' heads turned to watch him drive down the straight. The spectators should have been looking to their left, to watch him drive down the straight towards the bend but his subconscious mind observed that the mosaic of the spectators' heads looking down the track towards his car was missing. Fangio sensed he was being ignored; the spectators' attention was on something on the other side of the bend, which they could see from high up in the grandstand but Fangio, low down on the track, could not.

Once Fangio realised that the unusual pattern of the spectators' gaze had made him brake so hard he was able to use the information in his conscious mind whenever he raced at circuits with a blind bend.

Self-doubt

To recap, the RAS filter is responsible for filtering what remains unnoticed in our subconscious mind and what is allowed through into our conscious mind. When we experience difficulties and problems, the filter is usually set to allow the negative memories into our conscious mind. The positive experiences in our lives are just as real as the negative experiences but they simply don't have the same level of significance and therefore remain unnoticed. The more we filter out the positive memories and filter in the negative memories, the greater our levels of anxiety. If we constantly think negative thoughts, this is bound to affect our mood.

Negative DVDs are often memories of situations in which we struggle to cope. Continually replaying negative memories leads to higher levels of anxiety, which in turn can lead to self-doubt – the uncertainty that we will be able to successfully handle a difficult situation. I described this link between anxiety and self-doubt in Step 1, through the example of the Olympic gold medal-winning cyclist, Chris Hoy, who was plagued with anxiety in his early career. If Chris replayed the DVD memories of a poor race performance, the subsequent anxiety could lead him to doubt that he was good enough or that he would be able to live up to everyone's expectations.

Think of something that you're not very good at.

* ....

What DVDs come into your mind when you think about this?

* ....
* ....
* ....
* ....

If someone asked you to do something similar how would it make you feel?

* ....
* ....
* ....
* ....

How confident would you be about handling the situation successfully?

* ....
* ....
* ....
* ....

When they're first referred to me, all my clients are suffering from some kind of stress in their lives, which often causes either an anxiety disorder or depression. Not surprisingly, they often experience quite high levels of self-doubt, which affects their confidence. Sarah was involved in a car accident in which her granddaughter was injured. Sarah felt she was to blame (despite the insurance company's view to the contrary) and she completely lost confidence in her ability to drive. Another client, Peter, experienced high levels of anxiety over his heavy workload and an unsupportive boss that eventually led to him lacking confidence in his ability to make decisions at work.

The more negative DVDs that filter into our conscious minds, the more anxious we become about the difficulties in our lives. The increased anxiety leads to higher levels of self-doubt, which affect our confidence. If the cycle continues, eventually we succumb to anxiety disorders or depression. This cycle of vicious negative thinking can extend from the present into the future, so that we subconsciously contribute to our failures.

Self-fulfilling prophecies

If you believe it's going to be a disaster, you're probably right.

If we're feeling anxious or are in a depressed state, it's because our filters don't allow us to play a healthy mix of positive and negative DVDs. Instead, we constantly replay negative memories of the past and present. After a while, in our distressed state of mind, the filter lets through negative memories of the past and present so effectively that it starts to operate in the same way when it comes to playing DVDs about what the future might look like. Before we know it, we've started to think ourselves into failure.

A self-fulfilling prophecy starts when we begin to believe that we will fail in the future because we have lots of negative evidence to show us how we failed in the past. You might have responded similarly when I asked you to think about something you're not good at in the previous exercise. Anxiety and self-doubt negatively affect our confidence and begin to lead to an expectation of failure, which significantly reduces the chances of a positive or successful outcome. In effect, the additional anxiety produced by replaying negative memories of past failures increases our level of self-doubt to the point where we unconsciously self-sabotage our efforts, by doing things which are likely to increase our chances of failing.

The cycle of negative thinking

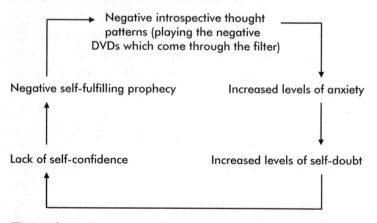

Figure 4

I was once asked to give a motivational talk to a group of thirty high-flying staff members in a global IT company. I'd been told that I could talk on any subject, so I decided to see if I could investigate the power of the mind to create negative self-fulfilling prophecies. I arrived early at the venue and laid the room out so that each table accommodated seven people. I had asked the organiser to ensure that each table had six high-fliers and a senior manager. The senior managers were there to observe the day and get to know the high-fliers. On each table I placed a plate, a cereal bowl, a bag of flour, a potato masher, a knife and a small coin. When everyone was seated I explained that I was a psychologist and that I wanted everyone to take part in an experiment. The reaction was varied – amusement, interest, discomfort and negativity registered on the faces of the members of the group. I explained that the senior managers would organise the experiment: they were to pour the flour into the cereal bowl and use the potato masher to pack it tightly. They should then turn the bowl upside down on the plate like a sandcastle, producing a flour 'pie', and place the coin on top.

Then, each of the six high-fliers would take it in turns to cut away a section of the flour pie, which would gradually become more and more narrow and increasingly less stable. The senior manager's job was to ensure each cut of the knife was a continuous movement from the top all the way to the plate. Anyone who didn't stick to this rule was ordered to take another cut. Eventually, inevitably, as one person started to cut a small piece of the flour pie, the coin would topple off the top. The forfeit for failure was that the person who'd made that fateful cut had to pick the coin out of the flour using only their teeth. Naturally, their face would become covered in flour.

I explained that we would run the experiment three times and that each time a participant dislodged the coin, they would be knocked out of the game for the next round. Although I was careful not to say this, in effect, each table of six high-fliers would eventually be left with three winners and three losers with flour on their faces!

I then asked the high-fliers to jot down their answers to the following questions *before* they took part in the experiment:

1 How appropriate did they feel this experiment was to a group of high-fliers in a blue-chip IT company, with 1 being 'very inappropriate' and 10 being 'very appropriate'?
2 How well did they think they would perform on this task, with 1 being 'not very well' and 10 being 'very well'?

3 How did they feel about the prospect of getting flour on
   their faces, with 1 being 'very uncomfortable' and 10 being
   'very unconcerned'?

I emphasised the importance of everyone being absolutely
honest about their feelings and reassured them that their answers
would remain anonymous. The participants put the piece of paper
with their answers in their pockets until the end of the experiment and we conducted the three rounds of the experiment.
Eventually, each table ended up with three winners and three
losers.

Everyone then took the piece of paper with their answers
out of their pockets. I asked those who had ended up with flour
on their faces to write 'L' on their paper, to signify they had
been a Loser. If they had evaded the floured-face embarrass-
ment, they were asked to write 'W' for Winner. The papers
were sorted into Winners and Losers and the average score for
each question for Winners v Losers calculated.

For question 1 – how appropriate was the activity, the
scores showed that the Winners were significantly more positive about the activity than the Losers – even before they began
the experiment.

For question 2 – how well did people think they would
perform, the scores showed that the Winners were slightly
more confident of performing well than the Losers – even
before they began the experiment.

For question 3 – how did people feel about the prospect of
getting flour on their face, the scores showed that the Losers were
very significantly more concerned about getting flour on their
faces than the Winners – even before they began the experiment.

It seemed the Losers were much less enthusiastic about
taking part in the experiment and far more anxious about the

threat of getting flour on their faces. This anxiety affected their levels of self-doubt, which translated into less confident knife-cuts. The more tense people were when cutting, the more likely they were to dislodge the coin and get flour on their faces by completing the forfeit of picking the coin up with their teeth.

The moral of the story is that if we fear a negative outcome, we can subconsciously contribute to increasing the likelihood of it happening. If our filter is programmed to spot all the potential negative outcomes of a situation, it's almost as if the body automatically works to deliver the programme accurately – we think ourselves into failing.

Thinking errors

To stop thinking ourselves into failure, we have to reset the filter, so that we play more positive memories to balance any negatives. Unfortunately, it's quite difficult to do this when we're experiencing high levels of anxiety. What keeps the filter in place so that the negative DVDs slip into our conscious minds? The answer is that we make 'thinking errors' or cognitive biases.[14]

Thinking errors are the negative assumptions about our world which, when we challenge them, often prove to be unfounded.

1 *All or nothing thinking* – things are placed in black or white categories. Anything short of perfection is viewed as a failure.
2 *Over-generalisation* – a single negative event is perceived as a never-ending pattern of defeat. The word 'always' is often used to describe negative events and 'never' to describe positive events.
3 *Disqualifying the positives* – positive experiences are described as not counting: 'it was easy, anyone can do that'.

4 *Jumping to conclusions* – negative interpretations occur even though there are no facts to support the conclusion: 'everyone's got it in for me today'.

5 *Magnification and minimisation* – magnifying your errors or other people's achievements. Minimising your achievements or other people's errors.

6 *Emotional reason* – assuming your negative emotions reflect the way things really are.

7 *Should statements* – directed at yourself, they encourage failure or defeat: 'I *should* have done this'. Directed at others, they encourage anger, frustration and resentment: 'you *should* have done that'.

8 *Labelling and mislabelling* – an extreme form of generalisation. Instead of describing an error, you attach a negative label to yourself or others: 'I'm hopeless', 'she is an idiot'. The language is often highly coloured or emotionally loaded.

9 *Personalisation* – seeing yourself or someone else as the cause of some negative external event over which you or the other person had no control.

David Burns did a wonderful job of identifying these errors.[15] He also identified another thinking error, which he called 'mental filter': 'dwelling on negative events to the exclusion of any positive events'. There seems to be a lot of overlap between Burns's mental filter and my explanation of how the RAS filter works. However, I believe it's incorrect to describe the RAS filter as a thinking error: thinking errors keep the filter in place, so that only negative memories consistent with the thinking error are allowed into the person's mind.

My client Paula was a good example of someone making multiple thinking errors. Paula was in her early forties, with two teenage daughters who both self-harmed (for no apparent reason, the girls inflicted cuts on their arms). Paula couldn't understand why they did this. Despite the best efforts of Paula and her husband, the girls refused to give any reasons for their behaviour, except to say that it had nothing to do with their parents. Paula said:

> I just can't understand it. The two of them are so stupid. They have everything they need: a nice house, loving parents, a decent standard of living. They're doing well academically and they have lovely friends. I feel like a complete failure. Other parents don't have this type of problem with their children. These days they never seem to be happy about anything, they're always arguing about something. Take Christmas Day, for example. We were just sitting down to watch the film in the evening when they ruined the whole day with their behaviour by starting an argument for no reason at all. Half an hour later, when I went to my younger daughter's bedroom, I found she'd cut herself again.

Poor Paula was understandably very anxious about the situation with her daughters, whom she clearly loved very much. But she wasn't helping the situation by making so many thinking errors.

Look back at the list of thinking errors and see how many thinking errors you can spot in what Paula said.

- ....
- ....
- ....
- ....
- ....
- ....

Paula and I identified these thinking errors:

The two of them are so stupid. Paula knew her daughters weren't stupid; both of them were very bright young women.

Paula was *mislabelling* them with her frustrations and by telling them they were stupid, was inflaming the situation. Paula rephrased her statement to reflect her view that their behaviour was destructive and didn't seem to make any sense.

I feel like a complete failure. This may have been another example of mislabelling but it was also an example of *magnification*. When we talked about Paula's role as a parent over the years, it became clear that the self-harm was relatively recent and that Paula had been very successful in many aspects of parenting.

Other parents don't have this type of problem with their children. This was an example of *emotional reason*. Paula may not personally know any parents who have similar problems but such parents certainly exist. Most teenagers go through a difficult patch and some choose extreme forms of behaviour during this time in their lives.

The children never seem to be happy about anything, they're always arguing about something. Paula recognised that this was an *over-generalisation*: there were lots of things they did take pleasure from and plenty of times when they didn't argue.

We were just sitting down to watch the film in the evening when they ruined the whole day. Paula was guilty of all or nothing thinking and disqualifying the positives. She later admitted that Christmas Day had, on the whole, been a pretty positive experience for the family. While her younger daughter had inflicted a minor cut on her arm, the whole day wasn't ruined.

Paula's multiple thinking errors allowed her filter to remain fixed, so that only the negative DVDs of Christmas Day made it into Paula's conscious mind. This was particularly true of the thinking error that her daughters were 'always arguing'. The more she replayed the negative memories of the arguments, the more anxious she became about the rows with her daughters.

Paula's increased anxiety was hardly surprising, as she'd noticed that rows often came before the incidents of self-harming. Her increased anxiety fuelled her feelings of self-doubt, which in turn led to a lack of confidence in her parenting ability, culminating in the description of herself as 'a complete failure'.

So, when her daughters began arguments, instead of remaining calm Paula allowed the anxiety, self-doubt and lack of confidence to combine, causing her to shout that her daughters were 'always arguing'. Her daughters responded by arguing passionately that this wasn't true, which Paula used to reinforce her thinking error: 'see, there you go again, always arguing!' Paula's behaviour contributed to creating the argument with her daughters, which increased the chances of them later self-harming. A negative self-fulfilling prophecy.

Paula wasn't responsible for her daughters' self-harming behaviour. That was clearly their choice. However, when Paula learned to challenge her thinking errors she filtered in positive aspects of her daughters' behaviour and consequently felt more positive about them. This meant she was able to deal with the arguments and rows more calmly, which reduced the likelihood of the consequent self-harming.

The exception to the rule – traumatic events

When we're struggling with challenging events and circumstances, we replay lots of negative DVDs, which increases anxiety and self-doubt. This affects our confidence and can lead to negative self-fulfilling prophecies. And when we make thinking errors, the RAS filter is fixed and allows a disproportionate number of negative memories into our conscious mind.

There is one exception to the rule about how our negative mind works: if we're unlucky enough to experience a traumatic event. As I wrote in Step 1, traumas are quite distinct from life events; everyone experiences life events but only some people are affected by trauma. Traumatic events are unusual, if not abnormal, experiences, such as abuse, serious criminal acts, major accidents or disasters. When we experience a trauma the mind often tries to protect us from its emotional consequences by not dealing with it. Instead of replaying the negative memory of the trauma over and over again, the filter seems to operate in reverse, by isolating the DVD on a high shelf right at the back of the library to try to make sure it never gets into the conscious mind. Short-term protection from a trauma can help keep us functioning but it can also prevent us from finding long-term solutions.

Louise, a client of mine, was in her early forties. When she was much younger, Louise had moved away from home to go to art college. While studying, she met Gary, a successful businessman quite a few years older than her. After a short romance, they decided to get married and moved into Gary's house, in a neighbourhood where many of his friends, family and work colleagues lived. For the first year of their marriage, everything seemed fine. However, one night Gary wanted to have sex but Louise felt too tired. Instead of acceding to Louise's wishes, Gary raped her. In the few months that followed, Gary raped Louise several times, sometimes quite violently.

Fortunately, Louise was eventually able to pluck up the courage to leave Gary and move back to her parents' house. She never told anyone what had happened. She didn't even acknowledge it to herself. She took the particularly painful memories of the rapes and isolated them on a high shelf at the back of the DVD library of her subconscious mind. If she never replayed those memories, she could pretend they didn't happen. This proved quite successful, up to a point; for the next twenty years she never once spoke about the rapes or acknowledged they had happened. However, unsurprisingly, she found it very hard to have relationships with men after what had happened with Gary. For many years, she simply didn't bother, fearing that a relationship might trigger distressing memories of the rapes.

When it seemed she had safely closeted the DVDs on their remote shelf, Louise started to engage in relationships again. However, she found it hard to experience the positive emotions of relationships and was unable to tell the men why she was finding it difficult to get emotionally close. Having to explain why meant acknowledging the existence of those painful memories. As a result, Louise often sabotaged her relationships: the closer she became to a man, the more likely she was to end the relationship or the more the man became frustrated with Louise's reluctance to become emotionally close, the more likely he was to end the relationship.

Then for some inexplicable reason, perhaps prompted by an unconscious trigger, Louise found herself blurting out her experiences of the rapes to a particularly intuitive close friend. Once the memories got through the filter, Louise found great difficulty in stopping them playing in her mind. Try as she might, she struggled not to replay the DVDs. Although she was sometimes able to control her thoughts during the day, she often had flashbacks in the form of nightmares when she had little power over her subconscious mind. Not surprisingly, she quickly became anxious, distressed and depressed.

During our sessions Louise worked very hard to come to terms with what had happened to her but it's a journey that's taken her almost twenty years. She now understands how her negative mind tried to cope with the trauma: her mind's short-term protection system prevented her from dealing with what happened to her and she was unable to move successfully on until she did. It's only by replaying the negative memories of a trauma that we are able to gain insights that allow us to face the negative emotions. If we balance this with replaying plenty of positive DVDs, we can come to terms with the trauma and eventually move on. Most people won't experience a trauma, however, if you need more information on trauma see our website www.mindhealthdevelopment.co.uk

Summary of Step 2

Negative thinking patterns can lead to us thinking ourselves into failure. By repeatedly playing only the negative DVDs that have been allowed through the RAS filter, our levels of anxiety increase, causing self-doubt to grow and diminishing our confidence, which can lead to negative self-fulfilling prophecies. The main reason for the filter being set to notice only negative memories is that we make thinking errors that keep the filter activated.

The exception to this rule is the way the mind tries to protect us from a traumatic event. After a trauma, the mind operates in a radically different way, refusing to replay the painful memories. This may have short-term benefits but can be psychologically damaging in the long-term.

The mind: the DVD library and the DVD player

The subconscious mind is the DVD library where memories are stored and the conscious mind is the DVD player. When we're worried, we replay negative memories related to our troubles.

The brain's filter

If the filter between our conscious and subconscious mind is set to notice negative memories, we replay a disproportionate number of negative DVDs.

Self-doubt

Replaying negative memories of situations where we struggled to cope causes anxiety and doubt in our ability to handle situations successfully, which affects our confidence.

Self-fulfilling prophecies

Negative self-fulfilling prophecies happen when we believe that we'll fail in the future because we replay lots of negative DVDs of how we failed in the past.

Thinking errors

Negative assumptions that we make about ourselves and others; thinking errors keep the RAS filter activated, so that we focus on negative memories.

The exception to the rule – traumatic events

When we experience a traumatic event the filter seems to operate in reverse, putting the DVD on a high shelf at the back of the library to try to make sure it never gets into the conscious mind.

In the next step I'll look at why we're all prone to the cycle of negative thinking and why some situations make this more likely than others.

STEP 3

Realise why you must accept yourself

Legend has it that, faced with difficult decisions, the Ancient Greeks consulted the Oracle in the Temple of Apollo at Delphi. On the wall of the temple was written, 'From the gods comes the saying: "know thyself"'.

Most psychologists agree that after a certain age, around our mid- to late twenties, we probably don't change much. We can be severely affected by significant emotional events such as traumas but even the changes these events cause seem transient. Eventually, we revert back to type. It's important to accept ourselves. No one's perfect, we all have strengths and we all have weaknesses; it helps our psychological well-being to maintain a healthy and balanced perspective.

'Why we must accept ourselves' is a very positive question. The better we know ourselves the easier it is to maximise our talents. The more time we spend doing what we have a talent for, the happier and more fulfilled we feel. Likewise, we get a poor return from investing hours of time trying to improve areas where we don't have much talent.[16] It's pretty soul-destroying to put in loads of effort to find we're only slightly better at the end!

The more time we spend in situations that play to our strengths, the more positive DVDs we'll record for the library of our subconscious mind. The more we replay those positive memories, the more confident we're likely to be. However, we all have our weaknesses and the more time we spend in situations where they are exposed, the more likely we are to be stressed, anxious or depressed.

The Human Factors Model

We all find certain situations stressful because of personal weaknesses. And there are common situations, such as a loved one's death, that everyone finds stressful, regardless of personal qualities. Either way, we're all likely to suffer from stress some time during our lives. The Human Factors Model helps to explain this. It's partly to do with the external world – the things that happen to us – and partly to do with our internal psychological make-up – how well each of us is equipped to deal with the external world. These two factors interact to determine our mood at a given moment: happy, confident, sad, anxious or depressed.

The external world

The external world is made up of three elements: life events, traumatic events and circumstances.

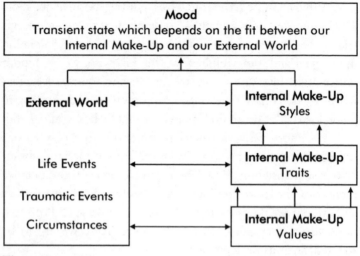

Figure 5

Life events

Whoever and whatever we are, we will all experience life events. The natural course of life brings events that can be psychologically challenging: the death of a close relative, changing jobs, illness or injury, the break-up of a relationship. Negative life events are normally external factors that cause us stress. Life events are inevitable, which is why we all suffer from the cycle of negative thinking at some time in our lives. I've worked with many people experiencing anxiety or depression as a result of difficult life events. In these instances it is relatively easy to pinpoint the source.

Stan was a man in his mid-forties coming to terms with impending blindness, a result of his diabetic condition. It's not hard to understand why he might feel depressed. However, some of the people I've worked with don't know what's causing their negative feelings; no obvious life event prompts their anxiety disorder or depression. The answer lies in the subconscious mind but the sufferer hasn't yet recognised it as the cause of their low mood. The person might be suffering many minor stresses, none of which on their own would be enough to cause depression.

My client Frances was experiencing symptoms of mild to moderate depression and couldn't put her finger on the reason. During our first session, she used the phrases 'a little', 'slightly' and 'a bit' to describe the negative things in her life. Frances was 'a bit fed up with work', 'a little worried about her health', 'slightly stressed by her teenage daughter' and 'a bit worried by her financial situation'. After a while, she realised that multiple minor life events were causing her depression. She acknowledged she could have handled any one of these minor events perfectly well but the cumulative effect of all four was causing the camel's back to break.

Traumatic events

Traumas are quite distinct from life events; they merit inclusion in the Human Factors model because they are part of some people's external world.

Circumstances

The third element of the external world is our circumstances, which may change from time to time and can make the effect of life events or traumas better or worse. For example, many people go through difficult and painful divorces but being affluent can cushion the effects. The famous entrepreneur, Duncan Bannatyne, noted after separating from his first wife that it was a lot easier going through a divorce when you had plenty of money to help you deal with the practical problems of running two homes instead of one.

Our finances are just one circumstance that can affect a life event or trauma. Family circumstances can also be crucial in determining how much support we get from our siblings or parents when we are faced with difficulties: an abused child who has a very loving and supportive family to whom they can turn will find this helps lessen the effect of the abuse. Geography can also play a part in determining how easy or difficult events are to cope with. I have many clients who are coping with elderly parents who are ill and in need of care. Generally speaking, the nearer they live to each other, the easier it is to successfully manage the situation. Levels of support at work can be a major contributor to worsening or lessening the effects of dealing with life events. Unsympathetic or unsupportive bosses and colleagues increase levels of anxiety for people already feeling stressed about coping with challenges.

Think of a minor or major life event you're going through at the moment.

- ....

Think about your financial, family, social and work circumstances: how have they made your current situation better or worse?

- ....
- ....
- ....
- ....

Internal psychological make-up

The interaction between our internal psychological make-up and our external world defines how well we will be able to deal with certain challenges: someone might cope very well with the break-up of a relationship but get very anxious and depressed at the thought of losing their job.

I like to describe this as 'pegs and holes'. Our external world is a constantly changing variety of holes and we are the pegs that have to fit into them. Naturally, we fit better into some holes than others. Our internal psychological make-up creates our unique peg shape. None of us are shaped to deal effectively with every life challenge we face but it's true to say that some people generally find it easier to cope than others. And once we reach our mid- to late twenties, our peg shape doesn't change much. This may help us to deal with certain aspects of our lives very well but may not help us to deal so effectively with other challenges. It's important to understand the different elements of our internal make-up.

Values

Our values – the beliefs we have about the world – form the base on which our internal make-up is built. They give us a code of acceptable conduct about how we should interact with people and society and are represented by the attitudes and behaviours that we strongly identify with, as opposed to the attitudes and behaviours we find unacceptable.

Where do our values come from? Usually, it's a combination of nature and nurture. We inherit some from our parents and some develop from the effect of the environment we live in. During our childhood and teenage years, our values continually evolve but by the time we reach our twenties, our values are relatively fixed and enduring. Later in life, we can be severely affected by significant emotional traumas but the changes these cause seem transient and eventually, we revert back to type.

On the whole, this is a very positive message, showing how resilient we can be.

Most of the time, we act in a way consistent with our values. Kelly was a woman brought up in the firm belief that we should always trust people and believe the best about them unless proved wrong. In some situations this is very desirable. Kelly was an excellent customer services manager, confident enough to delegate responsibility to her experienced staff, because she trusted them. Her staff members were also honest and trustworthy people; Kelly was a round peg in a round hole. Kelly's trusting nature brought out the best in the people she managed but in the wrong situation, it could be a real disadvantage. If she were required to manage someone dishonest or untrustworthy she would probably end up being taken advantage of: a round peg in a square hole.

Going back to your early years, what or who influenced your values?

- ....
- ....
- ....
- ....

What have been the most important lessons in life that you've learned and from where?

- ....
- ....
- ....
- ....

Are there any phrases that sum up your approach to life, where did they come from?

- ....

- ....
- ....
- ....

Traits

Traits include personality, such as introversion or extroversion; strengths[17] – the things we have a natural talent for, such as the ability to think analytically or bring harmony to a situation; and motivational, such as whether we are motivated by the promise of something good if we do it or the threat of something bad if we don't. As with values, our traits are more or less fixed by the time we reach early adulthood.

A range of psychometric tests exists to measure different personality traits. In Figure 6, a test score of four would suggest the person was moderately extrovert, tending to be outgoing and livelier in their behaviour than someone who is moderately introvert, perhaps with a score of seven. Even so, a person with a score of four is able to moderate their behaviour to the situation; if, for example, they were attending a funeral, they would act in a quieter, more restrained way. My colleague Craig is an extreme extrovert, scoring one on the scale. At a funeral, Craig finds it hard not to tell funny stories about the deceased person. Some people are offended by his behaviour, seeing it as inappropriate and disrespectful. In that situation, Craig is a square peg in a round hole. However, at a party he's seen in a very positive light: telling jokes and funny stories are seen as desirable – there, he's a square peg in a square hole.

Extroversion ◄――――――――――――――――――► Introversion

1----2----3----4----5----6----7----8----9----10

Figure 6

We all have a few traits that are very strong and less likely to be influenced by a situation. However, many of our traits are more moderate and allow us to adapt.

What are your strongest personality traits?

- ....
- ....
- ....
- ....

What do you have a talent for?

- ....
- ....
- ....
- ....

What motivates you?

- ....
- ....
- ....
- ....

Style

Our values and traits lead us to develop a certain style in the ways we typically behave. Style is how we display our traits and values: we can see and hear someone's style. Like values and traits, our style tends to settle by early adulthood. There are many measures of different styles, such as management style (the way we typically manage people) or conflict style (the way we typically try to deal with conflict).

Styles are defined by words that describe people's behaviour in certain situations. I worked with a woman in her sixties, Angela, who was described as having an 'authoritarian' management style.

Listening to her, it was easy to picture her barking out orders to her junior colleagues. Angela believed that this was the only way to make people perform tasks to her high standards. She told me she'd been sent on a management course to help her change her style, to become more democratic and collaborative in her approach, but she found it very hard to change. She was happy to deal with conflict directly; a strong aspect of her personality.

I asked Angela how appropriate it was to give someone a public telling-off if they made a careless error. She paused and shook her head slowly: 'Perhaps I'm just old-fashioned but I honestly believe that if someone has made a careless mistake they should be told in no uncertain terms about it – then maybe they'll be more careful next time.' In this situation, Angela's values revealed themselves in her trait for dealing with conflict very directly and were reflected in her authoritarian style. Angela's values, traits and authoritarian style weren't bad but unfortunately, they were deemed inappropriate by the company she worked for. She was a square peg in a round hole; something she found increasingly stressful. Unable to change her style to suit the situation, Angela eventually retired early, with the company's blessing.

Thinking about the way you behave most of the time, how would you describe your personal style?

* ....

If your best friend had to describe you in three words or phrases, what would they be?

* ....
* ....
* ....

Mood – a transient state

Mood is the result of the fit between our internal make-up and our external world. Mood isn't fixed, it is transient and constantly changes, depending on how we interact with the situations we find ourselves in. When we're the right shape peg for a hole, we feel confident and comfortable but if we're the wrong shape, we feel anxious, unhappy and uncomfortable. It's important to remember that mood is transient: even clinically depressed people aren't depressed all the time. Certain external situations, such as the death of a loved one, would affect most people negatively to some degree. Other external situations only affect us negatively if they clash with the internal make-up created by our values, traits and style. Some people enjoy deal-ing with conflict; other people hate it. As the proverb says, 'one man's meat is another man's poison'.

I spent some time working with John, who was experien-cing considerable stress in the new job to which he had recently been promoted. Promotion was a life event that ought to have been very positive for John; he'd worked hard for it. However, in the cut-and-thrust world of his industry, John had become the most junior person in a team whose culture encouraged managers to be openly critical of each other in meetings if things weren't going well.

John found this blunt environment bruising and difficult to work in. He came from a family where the values of being polite and treating people with respect were reinforced. In John's family, being strongly critical of people wasn't regarded as acceptable behaviour. The values of politeness and respect had translated into certain traits within John. He naturally wanted to keep the peace with others, rather than falling out with people, which was how he perceived the situation in management meetings. John's boss Paul took the view that: 'We're all big lads who can take it on the chin and dish it out in equal measure if there are problems with the business.' Paul seemed to enjoy conflict and thought it was healthy to have strong disagreements. After a few months, John began to feel very uncomfortable working in this environment and was aware that Paul was questioning his ability to participate effectively in management meetings.

John's values had influenced his traits, which had in turn influenced his natural style. Unfortunately, that style was regarded as ineffective in the management meetings. John was a square peg in a round hole and his mood was starting to suffer, as he felt increasingly stressed in meetings. He was filtering the negative memories of previous uncomfortable meetings into his conscious mind, which increased his levels of anxiety and he began to doubt his ability to operate effectively in meetings. As his confidence began to be affected, there was a danger that negative self-fulfilling prophecies about his ability were coming to fruition. John was making lots of thinking errors: 'I never seem to say the right thing in the meetings', 'the whole meeting was a disaster from start to finish'. The negative thinking cycle was starting to become well-established. Together, John and I recognised he had two options: to leave his round hole and find a square hole (either inside or outside his company) or to try to make his existing hole squarer, so it was a better fit. Potentially, John had a third option, to try changing his peg shape. However, given that our values, traits and styles are relatively enduring, there seemed little point in trying to change who he was.

Apart from management meetings, John enjoyed his work, so he decided to try to make the hole squarer. John accepted he wasn't like the other senior managers, because of his different values. He also accepted that he would only be able to operate effectively in meetings if he felt he was being true to his values. Fortunately, he had a strong background in finance and was very good with figures and data. By preparing thoroughly for the meetings, John could let his figures do the talking and use the data to draw conclusions in a less personal and direct manner. Rather than criticise the sales director for not achieving his targets, John used his data to ask some very polite but relevant questions: 'I notice from the figures that the average value of a contract sold this month seems to have fallen by 25% from the same month last year. What are the reasons and what plans are in place to rectify it?' This approach matched John's values but also reassured his boss that he was able to participate effectively in meetings.

The habits of unhappiness

Some people are more susceptible to psychological stress than others. I've noticed a pattern in many of the clients I've counselled: a high proportion have an internal make-up which results in them being more susceptible to psychological health problems. This susceptibility seems to be due to higher than average levels of threat sensitivity, where the filter is primed to allow negative DVDs into the conscious mind, which means that they are far more prone to negative thinking cycles.

Threat sensitivity

The first habit of unhappiness, threat sensitivity (which I mentioned briefly in Step 1), primes the filter to notice negative things through being exposed to at least one of three early life experiences: the effect of having threat sensitive parents, the effect of a life event that caused high levels of generalised anxiety and from which there was relatively little parental protection, or exposure to a traumatic event.

Children may inherit a genetic predisposition to threat sensitivity but threat sensitive parents are also likely to say things such as 'when you go out make sure you don't ...', 'be careful you always remember to ...' or 'I really wouldn't do that, it could be very dangerous to ...' Often, such statements are based on the parents' thinking errors and they reinforce the value that it's a scary world out there, full of potentially nasty, harmful people and situations that should be treated very carefully. Whether through the effects of nature, nurture or both, children become very threat sensitive.

Daisy was a classic example of someone who had been exposed to threat sensitive parenting and consequently suffered from psychological health problems later in life. Daisy worked as a client manager for an IT company. She had been there for several years and looked after one of the company's biggest accounts. The company's human resources manager referred Daisy to me for counselling after she had been ill with stress for several weeks as a result of the client director's (her boss) bullying of Daisy and some of her colleagues. Although the company had suspended the client director, they were very worried that Daisy would resign. The human resources manager was mystified why Daisy, of all the client managers, had succumbed to stress. Daisy was almost the perfect employee: she had been the company's most successful client manager for several years, she was well-liked by her colleagues and she was very conscientious in her dealings with both her clients and the support staff at head office. Despite all this, Daisy suffered from a chronic lack of confidence, which seemed to have been there long before the bullying client director had joined the company.

Where did Daisy's anxiety and self-doubt come from? When I started working with Daisy, she told me that she was the only child of older parents. Throughout her childhood, teenage and early adult life, Daisy's parents worried about everything she did and their worrying instilled a high degree of threat sensitivity in Daisy. When Daisy left school, she started teacher training but her parents were very worried that she wouldn't be able to cope with teaching unruly children and tried to persuade her not to become a teacher. Despite her parent's fears, Daisy spent several years successfully teaching at a primary school. Due to her success, the headteacher put a lot of pressure on Daisy to take on extra responsibility. Daisy felt that she was being bullied.

She spoke to her parents about the headteacher's pressure and told them she wanted to leave teaching to study for a Master's degree in business administration. Ironically, her worried parents tried to dissuade her from leaving the security of the teaching profession. The pressure from the headteacher eventually became too much and Daisy found the strength to go against her parents' wishes and leave teaching. Daisy gained her Master's degree and decided she wanted to follow a career in business. Yet again, her parents tried to talk her out of it, because they were worried she wouldn't be able to cope.

Throughout Daisy's life the influence of her parents' threat sensitivity reinforced Daisy's view of what a difficult and dangerous world she lived in. Her heightened levels of anxiety and self-doubt meant she lacked confidence and was very easily intimidated by authority figures such as the headteacher and the client director. Over the years, this resulted in several periods of sickness caused by stress and anxiety.

It's important not to take parental threat sensitivity out of context. Naturally, parents want to keep their children safe.

However, when parents continually send the negative message that it's a very dangerous world, this suggests to children that their parents have no confidence in their child's ability to deal with difficulties. My colleague Glyn has a great way of helping parents to assess risk: No Permanent Damage. If the risk of allowing a child to do something involves a fair chance of permanent damage, no parent ought to allow it. However, responsible parents should give their children the confidence to move outside their comfort zone by finding ways to help them identify and overcome minor risks.

The second type of experience that can lead to early life threat sensitivity in children is exposure to a life event that causes general anxiety. Delroy was a client who suffered anxiety disorders and bouts of depression throughout his adult life. When Delroy was eleven years old, his father had been diagnosed with cancer and over the following twelve months had been in hospital for long periods. Eventually, the cancer went into remission and although his father lived for many years, Delroy was constantly anxious the illness would return. His situation wasn't helped by the fact that he was an only child and felt he had to support his anxious mother during his father's lengthy stays in hospital. Delroy's filter became primed to notice the negative aspects of life: his increased threat sensitivity in childhood made him more prone to anxiety and depression in adult life.

The third type of experience underpinning early life threat sensitivity is where a young person has experienced a trauma. Cathy's sad childhood years paint a clear picture of how early life exposure to trauma can result in threat sensitivity. Cathy was seven years old when her parents split up. With no apparent warning, Cathy's mum left the family home to live with another man. Her dad found it very difficult to cope with Cathy and her younger brother Jeremy and they were often left to their own devices. After a few years, their father found a new partner, who didn't want anything to do with the children, so he decided they would be better off with their aunt and uncle. Cathy's aunt was a lovely woman, with no children; she treated Cathy and Jeremy as if they were her own. Cathy's uncle began to sexually abuse her when she was twelve years old and continued for many years. Cathy was continually let down by people that she should have been able to trust. Rejected first by her mother, then by her father, and abused by her uncle, it's not difficult to see how, from an early age, her filter was primed to look for the potential dangers in her world.

Parental threat sensitivity, general anxiety and traumatic incidents can all cause a young person to become threat sensitive, so that their filter becomes primed to let through negative memories. If a child is exposed to any of these experiences, they are likely to be more prone to psychological health problems later in life. Trauma in childhood is particularly likely to cause threat sensitivity.

Was your filter primed to notice negative things through early life experiences? If so, how has it affected you?

- ....
- ....
- ....
- ....

If you have children, or young nieces or nephews, how well do you manage the risk of being overly threat sensitive with them?

- ....
- ....
- ....
- ....

Pessimism

The second habit of unhappiness is pessimism. Playing negative DVDs of what the future might look like leads to pessimism: a belief that things can and will go wrong. Pessimism is linked to earlier death, poorer health (particularly psychological health) and less success in life. It seems that at work, at school and in sport, optimists stay with difficult and challenging situations, while pessimists don't do so well and often give up. A classic study shows this quite clearly. The subjects were life insurance salespeople, who work in a high-risk industry, where they frequently experience rejection and have a high drop-out rate but in which the rewards for those who succeed are high. The study found that optimistic sales people significantly out-performed pessimistic sales people.[18]

However, in some situations, pessimists out-perform optimists. I once worked with a human resources manager for the National Air Traffic Controllers' Association. She told me that while she liked most of the air traffic controllers individually, she noticed how negative and pessimistic they were as a group. Because pessimists are very good at spotting risks, they're likely to excel in roles such as air traffic control. In situations where the risk of something going wrong is small but the consequences are huge, pessimists perform better than optimists.

Optimistic salespeople and pessimistic air traffic controllers are useful illustrations of the Human Factors Model: square pegs for square holes and round pegs for round holes. We are who we are; if we accept ourselves, we can look for the situations in which we will excel and which will build our confidence.

In what situations do you find yourself being optimistic that things will turn out well?

• ....

- ....
- ....
- ....

In what situations do you find yourself being pessimistic that things will turn out badly?

- ....
- ....
- ....
- ....

Were your answers affected by things you have a talent or a lack of talent for?

- ....
- ....
- ....
- ....

Broadly speaking, it's an advantage to be optimistic, because optimists are less threat sensitive. However, blind optimism can get us into trouble. Blind optimism results from a refusal to recognise a difficult situation; burying one's head in the sand and hoping a negative situation will just go away (sometimes referred to as 'being in denial') can lead to psychological problems later on. If we're trying to deal with painful life events, it's important to face the brutal truth of the situation while at the same time remaining broadly optimistic that the situation will improve if we do the right things. This concept is often referred to as the 'Stockdale Paradox', after Admiral Stockdale, the highest-ranking US Naval officer to be captured by the North Vietnamese during the Vietnam War.

Stockdale was imprisoned for seven years in the notorious Hoa Lo prison: the 'Hanoi Hilton'. The prison regime was brutal: physical torture and solitary confinement in total darkness were common. Stockdale used his understanding of Stoic philosophy to help him survive but he noticed that some servicemen, when first captured by the Vietnamese, were unrealistically optimistic about how soon they would be released. This blind optimism resulted in their psychological health deteriorating very quickly as time passed and they remained imprisoned. Their initial confidence that 'we'll all be home by Christmas' was severely dented when Christmas came and went and they were still there. The servicemen who fared best were those who faced the brutal truth – that they wouldn't be home by Christmas or any time soon – but who also never stopped believing that they would eventually be reunited with their families.

This example demonstrates the importance of balance. If we are able to maintain a balance between optimism and pessimism, we can appreciate the sadness of difficult emotional situations yet become stronger for the experience. Although there may be professional advantages in being threat sensitive and pessimistic in jobs where being able to identify small but significant risks is important, these values and traits can be personally problematic.

Risk aversion

The pessimistic belief that things will go wrong is closely linked to the third habit of unhappiness, risk aversion, the aversion to taking chances or seizing opportunities. Unsurprisingly, risk-averse people are much less likely to take jobs where the risks – but also the rewards – are high, for example, sales jobs, where the basic salary is relatively small but it's possible to earn large bonuses.

How risk averse are you? Take this quick test to see. (This is not a scientific test!)

Look at the following questions and answer each one with O for Often, S for Sometimes and R for Rarely

1 How often do you take out insurance cover?
2 How often do you buy a lottery ticket or have a bet?
3 How often do you save money for a 'rainy day'?
4 How often have you changed jobs?
5 How often do you visit the doctor?
6 How often do you take part in challenging sports?
7 How often do you get your appliances serviced?
8 How often do you let your car's fuel gauge go down to 'empty'?
9 How often do you take preventive medicine?
10 How often do you make impulsive expensive purchases?

For the odd-numbered questions score 1 for O; 3 for S; 5 for R

- Q1 =   Q3 =   Q5 =   Q7 =   Q9 =   Total =

For the even numbered questions score 5 for O; 3 for S; 1 for R

- Q2 =   Q4 =   Q6 =   Q8 =   Q10 =   Total =
- Grand Total =

If your grand total was 10–17 you're probably risk-averse.
If you scored 18–25 you're probably moderately risk-averse.
Scores 26–33 suggest a balance between risk aversion and risk-taking.
Scores 34–41 suggest you're a moderate risk-taker.
If you scored 42–50 you're probably a risk-taker.

As with threat sensitivity and pessimism, it's important to recognise there is probably a healthy balance for risk. Highly risk-averse people may never leave the safety of their own front room; high risk-takers can end up regretting their actions.

The three habits of unhappiness often go hand in hand as part of our internal make-up. Threat sensitivity is a value, either instilled by parents or the consequence of a negative early life experience or trauma. Threat sensitivity leads to the trait of pessimism and is likely to be reflected in a risk-averse style of behaviour. Not everyone who has overanxious parents goes on to become threat sensitive. Not everyone who is exposed to generalised anxiety from a life event when they were relatively young develops pessimistic traits. Not everyone who experiences a trauma turns out to be risk-averse in later years. However, if you were unfortunate enough to have developed the habits of unhappiness early in life, you will be more likely to have a predisposition towards suffering stress, anxiety and depression.

The myth of weak character

Past a certain age, the fixed nature of our values, traits and styles reinforces the idea that some people, through no fault of their own, are less emotionally resilient than others. A person's ability to cope in difficult situations may be no more than an accident of birth. Those born into stable, positive families with relatively little early exposure to anxiety are simply more fortunate because they are less likely to be threat sensitive.

Although Admiral Stockdale coped better than other prisoners, it doesn't necessarily make him a 'strong' character and the other prisoners 'weak'. Stockdale's make-up was probably better suited to the situation; he may have come from a much more stable background than prisoners who coped less well. However, generally, we want to attribute a person's success or failure at coping with a particular situation solely to the individual, rather than accepting that the situation itself may have had a big part in deciding the outcome. Most people, placed in difficult, challenging situations, will respond in a broadly similar fashion; everyone will experience a degree of stress regardless of their internal make-up but a few will cope better than others.

Many people fall into the unhelpful and inaccurate trap of considering people who struggle with certain life events as weak and those who seem to cope well as strong. This is one of the reasons people suffering from psychological ill-health some-times get very little sympathy and are told to 'pull yourself together'. We can be guilty of assuming the main reason for their psychological problems is the anxious or depressed person's inability to cope with life. While their internal make-up plays a part, we shouldn't underestimate the difficulty of the external world they find themselves exposed to.

Psychologists call this tendency to attribute outcomes to the person rather than the situation Fundamental Attribution Error.[19] The fundamental error we make is to attribute the anxiety disorder or depression to the individual's internal make-up, rather than to life events, traumatic events or the circumstances of their external world. The Roman emperor Marcus Aurelius, who spent most of his life trying to turn back the barbarians from the Roman frontier, summed this up very well: 'Tell yourself each morning: today I shall meet an envious chap, an ungrateful one and a bully and if I had their life I could easily become one too.' Marcus Aurelius (like Admiral Stockdale) was a follower of Stoic philosophy, sometimes regarded as the early forerunner to cognitive behavioural therapy.

Do you remember Louise, who was raped by her husband Gary? How many of us made the mistake of questioning why Louise didn't leave Gary after he raped her the first time?

Surely a 'strong' character would have left Gary straight away? Such a conclusion would leave us guilty of making a fundamental attribution error. Louise was young, lived hundreds of miles away from her parental home, was married to an older, very successful, man and lived in his house, with lots of his friends, colleagues and family close by. The rape left her emotionally hurt and confused. Many women, like Louise, abused physically, sexually and emotionally within what appears to be a stable relationship, often endure such abuse for years. The situation such people find themselves in, rather than their weakness, results in their staying in the relationship.

Summary of Step 3

Once we reach our mid- to late twenties, we don't change much, so we must accept ourselves for who we are. As the message at the Temple of Apollo said: 'know thyself'.

We all find it difficult to deal with certain life events, such as the death of someone we love, regardless of our internal make-up. Depending on our make-up, we all find some events easier to deal with than others (think pegs and holes). Some people, because of their make-up, find it generally harder to deal with difficult events. These people, through no fault of their own, are more susceptible to stress, anxiety and depression.

If we understand how the relationship between our internal make-up and the external world can lead to the negative thinking cycle that causes anxiety disorders or depression, we can begin to move forward. Understanding ourselves, recognising our strengths and weaknesses and accepting ourselves for who we are will help us to have a balanced view. This is the cornerstone of healthy self-esteem and a valuable step in changing our lives from within.

The Human Factors Model

The Human Factors Model attempts to explain how our internal psychological make-up interacts with our external world. It helps us to understand why we find some events more difficult and challenging than others.

External world

The external world is made up of three elements: life events, traumatic events and circumstances.

Internal psychological make-up

Our internal psychological make-up has three elements: values, traits and styles. These elements make us who we are.

Mood – a transient state

Mood is the result of the fit between our internal make-up and our external world.

The habits of unhappiness

Threat sensitivity, pessimism and risk-aversion all make people more susceptible to psychological ill-health.

The myth of weak character

Generally we want to attribute a person's success or failure in coping with a particular situation to the individual rather than the situation.

STEP 4 ✖

Master the use of your positive mind

This step has some simple exercises and techniques that will have a significant impact on your ability to challenge thinking errors and enable you to use your positive mind.

Practice makes permanent

Most forms of mental health problems result from our filter being set to notice negative memories, which increases anxiety and self-doubt, decreases confidence and can lead to negative self-fulfilling prophecies – the negative thinking pattern. But it's important not to get carried away. Playing occasional negative DVDs is quite normal and can help us deal with difficult situations. Psychological health problems begin when negative thinking patterns become unbalanced and habitual, which is why threat sensitivity, pessimism and risk aversion are described as the 'habits of unhappiness'.

This step is about how to consciously challenge the thinking errors that cause the filter to feed us a stream of negative memories. Only by using the positive mind to continually challenge thinking errors can we reset the filter. If we stop challenging the thinking errors, the filter will slip back into place and block out the positive DVDs. It's like physical training: if we don't make the effort to get some regular exercise, we soon turn into couch potatoes. It's the same with the mind. If we don't make the effort to use the positive mind regularly, we get into unhealthy thinking habits that make us mentally unfit.

The graph of success isn't a straight line upwards. The exercises and techniques in this book take a little time to work; on average, six weeks of regular practice for at least ten minutes a day (although this depends on the severity of the thinking errors). You'll have good days and bad days but the bad days don't cancel out the good days. The good days still happened and the positive DVD memories prove it! I liken the bad days to how some people react when they're on a diet. My client Sue often went on diets to lose some weight. She'd do well for a couple of weeks, gradually lose a few pounds, and then have a bad day when she ate lots of junk food. Instead of accepting that it was just 'one bad day' and returning to healthier eating the next day, Sue would abandon the diet completely and continue her unhealthy eating habits. The bad days don't cancel out the good days.

It's important to remember this isn't about changing who you are as a person. To a large degree, it's the opposite: it's about accepting who you are but trying to change your perception of life. Sometimes the changes required are relatively minor. Often it's no more than noticing the positive things that already exist in our external world.

Good things are around us all the time but when we feel anxious or depressed, our filters simply don't allow the good things to make it from the subconscious to the conscious mind. The wonder of nature, small acts of kindness, beautiful music, good food, children's laughter, overcoming life's little challenges, church bells, a person's touch – all can go unnoticed if we let them.

Stop reading for a moment and look around you – what good things can you see, hear, feel, smell or taste?

- ....
- ....
- ....
- ....

Well-formed outcomes

This exercise is designed to help your positive mind clarify what you want to achieve in the longer term. Research shows that the most successful therapists ask their clients to define precisely what it is that they want from counselling: to develop well-formed outcomes (WFOs).[20]

Clearly defining what outcomes we want helps us achieve two things. First, it helps us to think about what's missing from our lives. Second, when we've identified what we want it's easier to stay motivated when the going gets tough. Have a go at creating some WFOs by answering these seven questions.

1 What outcomes do you want to achieve?

This is a very broad question but the greater the clarity the better. There are no right or wrong answers. Think about what's missing from your life – what would make you happier?

- ....
- ....
- ....
- ....

2   Where, when and with who do you want to achieve your
    outcomes?

Sometimes the problem is related to a certain aspect of our
lives. There might be a particular time when the problem occurs
or a period in which you need to achieve your outcomes. Or
the outcome might involve specific people. Identifying these
constraints can help you focus.

- ....
- ....
- ....
- ....

3   What will it look, sound and feel like when you've achieved
    your outcomes?

Such visualisation can be very important in motivating yourself
when the effort seems too much. Having an attractive picture
of what the future holds if the outcomes are achieved spurs
most people on.

- ....
- ....
- ....
- ....

4   What do you need to change and what do you need to accept
    to help achieve your outcomes?

This is potentially a difficult question but it throws some
light on what you can and can't control and where you should
channel your energies.

- ....
- ....
- ....
- ....

5 Will you lose anything if you succeed in achieving your outcomes?

There are, potentially, losses in achieving outcomes. From a psychological perspective, people might worry about losing their depression or anxiety because they will no longer have an 'excuse' for not doing certain things. Sometimes the losses are more tangible: I've worked with people who have been trying to resolve troubled relationships or difficulties with regard to their job. To achieve their outcomes they may need to lose the relationship or the job.

- ....
- ....
- ....
- ....

Loss aversion (fear of losing something we value) and commitment (the amount of effort we have already put into something) are powerful factors behind our occasional irrational behaviour. Sometimes, they cause us to stay in doomed relationships or continue in a job that makes us miserable. If we take a long-term perspective, it can help us get over the idea of short-term loss. If levels of commitment to a job or relationship are making us behave irrationally, it can help if we look at the situation here and now. Would we jump into this relationship or job if we were starting afresh? Potential losses have to be weighed against potential gains.

6 Is the outcome worth the effort and what type of effort are you going to have to make?

If the outcome doesn't seem worth the effort, you need to ask yourself some more questions. Are you really clear about the potential positive benefits of making the changes in your thinking? Do you understand the potential negative long-term consequences of not changing your thinking? If the answer to this question is a definite: 'Yes. The outcome is worth the effort', don't cheat on how much honest effort you put in. What kinds of effort will you have to make?

- ....
- ....
- ....
- ....

7   What will be the positive consequences of achieving your outcomes?

List as many benefits as you can that will come from being able to use your positive mind to notice the good things about you and your life. This may overlap with some of the other questions but that's a good thing. It reaffirms what you already know – that the outcome will be worth the effort!

- ....
- ....
- ....
- ....

One of my clients, Alex, was a nurse who had worked for eleven years in the busy accident and emergency department of a large inner-city hospital. Alex had experienced a number of life events within six months. Her relationship, which had lasted seven years, had ended and her ex-partner had left her with some financial problems. She had suffered three bereavements: an uncle, her grandmother and a close work colleague. She described the combination of these events as 'robbing her of the ability to cope with life'.

Before this, Alex described herself as 'resilient'. As a result of the life events, she experienced various problems: difficulty sleeping, feeling very lethargic, crying for no apparent reason, an inability to concentrate at work and being short-tempered with colleagues and patients. Work had been the major stabilising influence in her life but she was experiencing panic attacks and having difficulty making decisions as the anxiety and self-doubt began to creep in. Alex's manager noticed her problems and suggested she take some time off work to seek help. She'd been to see her GP, who prescribed mild antidepressants and referred Alex to me for counselling. At our first session, I set Alex the task of writing her WFOs as her homework. This is what she produced.

1 What outcomes do you want to achieve?

I want to get better, feel normal not depressed, I want to feel happy and stop crying. I want to be able to do my job as well as I used to, I want to get back to being Alex. I want to manage my stress and anxiety and increase my self-confidence. I want to be less selfless, I want a balance between caring for other people and caring for myself, I'd like to be able to talk openly about my feelings.

It's easy to see the self-doubt and lack of confidence that has crept into Alex's mind from the anxiety of viewing lots of negative DVDs. These affect her ability to do her job 'as well as I used to'. Many of the things Alex mentions are typical – the desire to get back to where she was before she became depressed is very common. However, some of the things she mentions are about taking herself on a positive journey beyond getting 'back to being Alex'. Talking openly about her feelings is something that Alex didn't previously do.

2 Where, when and with who do you want to achieve your
   outcomes?

   Now, as soon as possible! Over time I would like to be able to
   balance the good days with the bad days both at work and in
   my home life. I realise this will take a little time but I hope to
   achieve this in a few weeks with the help and support of my
   manager and my counsellor. I've also realised that the most
   important person in achieving my outcomes is me – I need
   to change my thinking.

Like many people, Alex wants a quick end to her stress and anxiety but realises that changing her way of thinking will take a
while. Given that she's been struggling for about six months, a
few weeks isn't an unreasonable time in which to challenge her
thinking errors and reset her filters. Alex also realises that
although she will benefit from my support and the help of her
manager, achieving her outcomes is down to her.

3 What will it look, sound and feel like when you've achieved
   your outcomes?

   I will be able to see and clarify exactly what is stressing me
   and I will be able to hear my own needs. I see myself dealing
   effectively and managing a range of stressful situations both
   at home and in my work. I will feel very balanced in the way
   I am dealing with problems. I am neither panicking nor pre-
   tending they don't exist. I will have got my confidence back
   and will be able to make decisions more easily. I will feel
   calmer and more relaxed; life will have slowed down so that
   I can take each situation in my stride.

Alex is clearly able to visualise what success looks, sounds and
feels like. When I asked her for more detail she was able to give
me specific examples, particularly for her work.

4 What do you need to change; and what do you need to accept
   to help you achieve your outcomes?

   I need to take charge of my life. I need to be more honest
   with myself. I know that sometimes I give up too easily. But
   on other occasions I bang my head against a brick wall and I
   have to accept that there are some things I can't control.

Alex's response to this question is fairly typical. I was able to
help her to be more specific about what she could control and
what she had to accept.

5 Will I lose anything if I succeed in achieving my outcomes?

   My sanity if I don't! I will lose some of my selflessness. Will
   I become more selfish? I will lose my self-doubt and become
   confident but does confident mean arrogant? Will I become
   an arrogant fool who people don't like?

Alex clearly recognises that she needs to achieve her outcomes
to become well again but her self-doubt comes through in her
response to this question. She doesn't want to be seen as selfish
or arrogant but from her previous answers it's clear she understands that the balance needs to shift more towards addressing
her needs. It's worth mentioning that many people who suffer
from psychological health problems find it difficult to get a balance between selflessness and selfishness.

6 Is the outcome worth the effort and what type of effort are
   you going to have to make?

   Ultimately yes but it's going to be a lot of hard work. I know
   I'll have to regularly attend my counselling sessions and do
   all the homework if I'm going to get better.

Alex wasn't kidding herself about the amount of effort required
to change her thinking. She clearly understood that she had

to make the effort. This links to the point she made in her answer to question 2: 'I've also realised that the most important person in achieving my outcomes is me – I need to change my thinking.'

7 What will be the positive consequences of achieving my outcomes?

I will feel well. I will not be an inconvenience to others, which is how I feel at the moment. I think my personality may change a bit. I will become a more balanced person. I will see the benefits in my relationships at work and in my personal life. I will like myself more. I will have the confidence to develop my career and I will be more confident in relationships in the future.

This response gave us the opportunity to discuss what Alex needed to accept about herself: that certain, fairly well-established aspects of her personality, wouldn't change. We were also able to talk about how she could change the perception both of herself and the way she responded to certain situations.

There are no right or wrong answers in WFOs. Completing yours is an opportunity to explore your thoughts and feelings. The more effort you put into this exercise, the more helpful you'll find it.

• **Tip:** *Use prompts to help your motivation.* Once your WFOs have helped you to identify what you want, use photographs, little notes or even posters featuring something very positive as visible reminders. Sue, my client who often went on diets to lose some weight, had a number of problems that led to a lack of confidence. Being overweight was one of these issues. Sue's WFOs included looking fitter, healthier and weighing less. On her fridge, Sue stuck a photograph taken on holiday in the Bahamas several years ago, when she was at her ideal weight. The photo helped motivate her to stay on track with her diet.

- **Tip:** *Use the power of occasional negative thinking.* Sometimes we can use the negative memory of an outcome we want to avoid to help motivate us to make the right choices. Sue could have used a photograph of herself looking very overweight as a negative thought to help her not to stray from her diet.

The positive list

Although occasional negative thoughts can be useful it's important not to dwell on negative thoughts too often. People experiencing stress, anxiety disorders or depression are out of the habit of replaying DVDs that make them feel happy. By consciously creating a list of positive memories, we can remind ourselves of some of our favourite happy memories.

Writing a list of positive memories is a very simple, but effective, exercise. The list can include anything that makes you smile or feel happy when you replay it: friends and family who love you, activities you enjoy, your achievements, qualifications or talents, interesting experiences, wonderful days out, memorable holidays, meaningful pieces of work – anything that makes you feel positive. As with WFOs, there are no right or wrong answers.

Some examples positive DVD memories that people have shared with me include: the day I got married, my three children, planting flowers in my garden, my cat, taking a hat trick in a cricket match when I was eighteen, swimming with dolphins, John Wayne films, going for lunch with my best friend at our favourite restaurant, running the London marathon, a good back massage, securing a successful business deal, my partner's smiling face, going for a drink with friends after work, eating a bacon and tomato sandwich while reading the *Racing Post* on a Saturday morning, being on the beach with my kids, the day I got my degree, watching my team win the FA Cup Final, buying my house and making it into a home, a really good cup of coffee, walking my dog in the countryside, cooking Christmas dinner for the family.

I've noticed that it's very common for people to list the significant positive life events, such as getting married or the birth of their children. However, it's always a good sign when people recognise that small things can give them joy – like a 'really good cup of coffee'. If you're lucky, you'll only get married once but you can have the pleasure of a good cup of coffee every day of your life! Noticing the small positive things that occur each day is one of the most important changes we need to make in our thinking patterns.

- **Tip:** *Do it a little at a time.* If you feel overwhelmed by the idea of coming up with a list of positive memories, keep this book by your bed and jot down two or three positive memories every night. There are benefits to doing the exercise this way: first, it's easier to do the exercise in bite-sized chunks; second, the effect of doing it each day starts to become habit-forming and third, playing positive DVDs last thing at night can be a pleasant way to drop off to sleep and, because we are more in tune with our subconscious mind during sleep, can also lead to sweeter dreams!
- **Tip:** *Go from the general to the specific.* Think of general things first and develop them into specific examples later. It might be easier to think of 'my home' as a general positive, which you can later develop into 'sitting in front of my fire on a cold winter night with a cup of hot chocolate'. Developing detailed memories engages all five senses, which helps the

parasympathetic nervous system to get the neurotransmitters flowing so that you start to feel good.

- **Tip:** *Don't prioritise.* It makes the task harder if you try to think of the most positive events in your life in order of rank and can block your thinking. Ray told me how he got stuck on this exercise when he felt he had to put the day he got married as his 'number one'. He thought if his wife read the list and found their wedding wasn't right at the top, she would be very hurt. Although his wedding day was a positive memory, it wasn't the most positive in his life. After explaining how important it was not to prioritise, Ray put his wedding at the head of the list and moved on easily, in the knowledge that the order wasn't important.
- **Tip:** *The treasure hunt.* Laura was a very successful accountant, suffering from a deep-seated depression that had been with her for years. Laura felt she was a failure and that her work was worthless. Much of Laura's problem stemmed from the fact that she was starved of love and affection as a child. She was rarely given any positive reinforcement about anything she achieved and was occasionally beaten by her parents when she failed to live up to their expectations. Her father made it clear to Laura that he would have preferred a son to a daughter. When I asked Laura to complete her positive list she found it almost impossible. She told me that when she tried to do it her mind locked down and refused to play any positive DVDs. I asked Laura to go on a treasure hunt around her house and find objects or memorabilia that triggered positive memories. Laura brought several items to our next session: a pair of earrings from her daughter, an old ticket stub from a school visit to a West End musical, a photograph of her family and a CD of punk music from her days at college. These items triggered very positive memories for Laura, which she was able to add to her list.

The point of creating the list is to deliberately get you back into the habit of thinking positively. By trawling the shelves of your memory library, you can use your positive mind to challenge thinking errors, shift the filter and push the positive memories from the subconscious into the conscious mind. Writing a list of positive memories helps us, literally, to see our life through a different filter. Our anxiety levels and self-doubt decrease as we replay the memories of enjoyable activities for which we have a talent. Our confidence starts to return when we think of our achievements and qualifications. We begin to like ourselves more and our self-esteem improves as we relive the memories of spending time with family and friends with whom we have mutual love and respect.

When you're ready, make a start on your positive list and continue it later.

- ....
- ....
- ....
- ....

Eventually, most of the people I work with manage to come up with a list of very effective positive memories. However, they often note that these are memories of the past rather than recognition of the present. Creating a positive list is a good exercise but we need to take it a stage further; to practise looking for positive DVDs in the present. If we can do this, we can start feeling more optimistic and hopeful, not only about the present but also about the future.

Keeping a diary

The next stage is to become more consciously aware of your thoughts by keeping a diary. Like creating a positive list, it's best done regularly, at the end of the day. Completing exercises regularly helps make your positive thinking more systematic and habitual. Remember, practice makes permanent.

Keeping a diary is quite simple: at the end of every day write down a few sentences to describe what has happened, then rate the day between '1 – it was a terrible day' and '10 – it was a fantastic day'. Check what you've written to see if you're making any thinking errors, particularly if you gave the day a low score. By challenging your thinking errors, you question the negative assumptions they're based on and when the assumptions are proved false, your score for the day will often improve.

Recording your thoughts and feelings every day is not only a powerful way of challenging your thinking errors, it also allows you to compare days. You can track patterns to see whether there are certain triggers that cause you to score some days higher or lower than others. If your scores are consistently low, this may be due to certain thinking errors locking your filter so the positive memories of the day are prevented from entering your conscious mind.

Martin came from a large family of seven brothers and sisters. He was experiencing a number of difficult life events: one of his brothers had died unexpectedly, his sister was seriously ill, his relationship had recently ended and he'd been involved in a car crash, which had rocked his confidence. Martin didn't have a little rain falling into his life – he had a monsoon! After creating his WFOs and positive list, I set Martin the task of keeping a diary and scoring each day. At our next session, Martin recalled a particularly low-scoring day that he'd rated as a 2. He felt stressed at work, he was unable to concentrate because he kept thinking about his sister's illness and he was worried about the fact that he had to drive to a sales meeting near to where he'd crashed his car. When he got home in the evening, he had a difficult phone call from his brother's widow about some legal issues that had arisen because his brother had died without making a will. Martin also wrote in his diary how he felt sad that he no longer had the emotional support of his partner.

Martin felt thoroughly depressed and his rating for this particular day summed it up. I noticed that Martin's diary didn't mention what he'd done after his sister-in-law's phone call. When I asked him, Martin closed his eyes and started to search for the memory. After he'd located the DVD in his mental library he nodded his head and then smiled, as it passed through the filter into his conscious mind and he started to replay it. 'I remember now. I went to church – I sing with a gospel choir and it was our night for choir practice. I enjoyed the singing and a few of us went for a drink and a meal afterwards.' I asked Martin why he hadn't written that in his diary. His reply was, 'Well, somehow it didn't seem to count.' Further gentle probing revealed that Martin felt it was 'wrong' to acknowledge anything positive in his life because he had to focus on the difficult negative events he was dealing with, particularly his brother's death. I asked Martin to reassess the day. He thought for a while and eventually said: 'Well, taking the evening into account as well, the day as a whole would have rated about a 5.' A much more balanced score.

Keeping a diary is excellent practice for challenging thinking errors. To paraphrase Shakespeare, 'no day is a bad day but thinking makes it so'. Even on our most difficult days good things happen but they often get filtered out. If we reset the filter, the good things are noticed. When we notice the good things, this improves the way we rate the day.

- **Tip:** *Remind yourself.* If you're having difficulty resetting the filter because you're still making thinking errors, ask a family member or a friend to point them out to you. For example, I'm prone to making 'should' statements; Glyn helps me challenge these by pointing them out.

- **Tip:** *Capture the moment.* Try to find a few minutes each day to capture the moment: admiring a glorious sunrise, watching your children play or looking at a beautiful building. Stop what you're doing and mentally 'record' the moment in every detail. Then add it to your diary entry at the end of the day.
- **Tip:** *Pleasure v effort.* Even on difficult days, where there hasn't been much to enjoy, challenging your thinking errors may help you realise that you've still achieved a lot. Score the day on how much effort you put in, rather than just how pleasurable it was.
- **Tip:** *Write something positive every day.* On a bereavement counselling course I met Mary, who carried a lovely notebook in which she recorded inspirational sayings, proverbs, thoughts, quotes and prayers. She told me that whenever she felt down, she only had to read a couple of pages from her book and she felt her mood lift. You could write something positive every day in your diary or, like Mary, keep a separate notebook. Here's a thought to start you off: 'If you can enjoy the simple pleasures in life, you'll rarely be disappointed.'

Think of a few of your favourite phrases or sayings:

- ....
- ....
- ....
- ....

Plus 4s

Sometimes it can be quite difficult to eject a negative DVD from our conscious mind once it's taken hold. In these circumstances, it's hard to change our perception of the day just by playing the positive memories. The way to overcome this is to use distraction; doing things often distracts the mind from our troubles. I ask my clients to take part in at least one of four specific activities *every day*. I call these activities the 'plus 4s'. Adding these to your day will mean you have something positive to focus on when you write your diary.

Mini-projects

Set yourself a small project that has obvious results when it's finished: clear the spare room, tidy the garden, mend something that's broken, wash the car or defrost the fridge. The task doesn't have to be enjoyable but it needs to be something that will give you a sense of satisfaction when it's finished. A project that lasts no more than an hour works best: it's big enough to give a sense of satisfaction but not so big that you're tempted to put it off. If you want to work on something bigger, break it down into bite-sized chunks and define success as completing a chunk.

Write down a few projects or tasks that need doing:

* ....
* ....
* ....
* ....

Phone a friend

Put some effort into a relationship with someone who you care about. Phone a friend you haven't spoken to for a while or invite them round for a cup of tea. Send a family member a text message or a postcard. Buy someone flowers for no special reason, just to let them know that you are thinking about them.

Good friendships are important: people who attempt suicide are more likely to be seriously ill, to be unemployed and to have poor relationships with their friends and family.[21]

Who are the people that are important to you? What small gestures would improve your relationship?

- ....
- ....
- ....
- ....

Altruistic acts

Do something for someone else. Small acts of kindness for which you've had to 'put yourself out' are a good way to feed your self-esteem. Mow your neighbour's lawn, look after a friend's children, visit someone in hospital, help a charity or donate blood. Sometimes we feel even better when we've done something for someone without them realising.

What could you do to help someone in the next few days?

- ....
- ....
- ....
- ....

Proper selfishness

Do something you really enjoy that you've neglected for a while. Or take up something new that you've always wanted to do. Read a book, go to the gym, have a long soak in the bath, listen to your favourite music, enrol in a language class or join a sports club. People suffering from anxiety or depression often stop taking part in activities that they enjoy but these kind of things are another way to create positive memories.

What activities might you enjoy spending some time doing?

- ....
- ....
- ....
- ....

Making sure we've completed at least one Plus 4 activity every day is another way of using our positive mind. It systematically challenges thinking errors, because it ensures we'll have at least one positive DVD to play at the end of the day. The more positive memories we've recorded and replayed during the day, the less anxious we feel. As anxiety recedes, self-doubt decreases and confidence begins to improve, which leads us into positive self-fulfilling prophecies. The two factors that combine to produce a depressed state of mind are negative introspective thinking patterns and a decline in participation in activities, particularly pleasure-giving activities. Plus 4s help address both these factors.

The gratitude list

The gratitude list, or to put it more simply, 'counting our blessings' is a great way to challenge all or nothing thinking, disqualifying the positives and magnification and minimisation. When they first come to see me, many clients find it difficult to express any gratitude for the good things in their lives. They feel guilty about being in a negative mood when they know there are people who are less fortunate. However, once they've started to learn the steps for changing their lives from within they find that consciously being grateful is a wonderful way to stay psychologically healthy. The less gratitude we experience in life, the unhappier we are likely to be.[22] This shouldn't come as any surprise: it's quite logical – the more we have to be thankful for in our lives the happier we'll be. The key is recognising it. Writing down the things in life that we're grateful for is a powerful tool to help us to use our positive mind.

The gratitude list is subtly different to the positive list. Whereas the positive list involves replaying specific memories, the gratitude list may include broader concepts, such as good health or being employed. Gratitude often, though not always, involves comparisons with those less fortunate – it stops us taking the good things in our lives for granted.

What are you grateful for in your life?

* ....
* ....
* ....
* ....

* **Tip:** *Create your own phrase.* A neat phrase can help remind you of everything you have to be grateful for. My favourite phrase came from a DJ on Sting FM, a black music station in Birmingham: 'Too blessed to be stressed'. When I feel a little bit down I replay that phrase in my head and it triggers many positive memories.

Visualisation

Keeping a diary, doing Plus 4s and writing a gratitude list all help us use our positive mind to systematically challenge thinking errors so that we can adjust the filter to allow the positive DVDs to flow into our conscious mind. Visualisation is a powerful technique for enhancing the memory, so that it becomes easier to recall and more effective in changing our mood. Visualisation involves replaying the DVD and using all the senses to enhance the memory. If we were using a memory of walking along the beach, we could bring to mind what we would see, hear, feel, smell and taste: the blue sky, the sound of the waves, the warmth of the sun on the skin, the smell of the salt water and the taste of an ice cream.

Think of a really positive, happy and fulfilling memory that, if enhanced, would build your confidence. You may be able to use something from your positive list. Use all your senses to help you relive the experience:

What can you see? (people, buildings, plants, colours, shapes, fine detail)

- ....
- ....
- ....
- ....

What can you hear? (voices, laughter, music, birdsong, loud, soft, gentle, strong)

- ....
- ....
- ....
- ....

What can you feel? (texture, heat, cold, touch, emotions)

- ....
- ....
- ....
- ....

What can you smell? (perfume, cooking aromas, flowers)

- ....
- ....
- ....
- ....

What can you taste? (sour, sweet, bitter – link with smell and feel)

- ....
- ....
- ....
- ....

By replaying the DVD repeatedly we increase its effectiveness at making us feel happy, relaxed and confident. We can also 'anchor' the positive memory and its accompanying positive feelings to a spoken word and a physical gesture. For example, at the end of replaying a positive DVD of walking along the beach, you might gently squeeze your little finger and say the word 'sunshine'. If you practice anchoring the word and gesture to the feelings you experience when you replay the memory of the beach, after a while, just squeezing your finger and saying 'sunshine' will be enough to recreate the positive feelings.

I used visualisation and anchoring very effectively with Steven, an administrator at a financial services company, who had been through a difficult separation from his wife and young daughter. He also had problems at work, from an aggressive manager, Patricia. Whenever Steven had disagreements with her, his confidence hit rock bottom. He felt so down that he visited the occupational health manager, who gave him sick-leave and referred him to me. Over the next few weeks, Steven worked through his WFOs, positive list, diary and Plus 4 exercises. He was almost ready to return to work on a gradual rehabilitation programme but the thought of having to work with Patricia still caused him great anxiety. To combat this we used a visualisation technique (described later) to enhance a positive DVD and improve his confidence in stressful situations with Patricia.

Steven had previously served in the Navy as a medical orderly. He had seen active service, successfully treating wounded servicemen in very stressful combat conditions. We used his memory of remaining calm and confident while treating injured servicemen as his ship was being attacked by enemy aircraft. He created an anchor from the phrase 'action stations' and the gesture of rubbing the back of his neck. On his first day back at work Steven had to attend a meeting with Patricia. He later told me that as he sat down he felt his anxiety level rise and he was worried he might start to panic. He began to rub the back of his neck gently and mentally said 'action stations'. This triggered the positive memory and the accompanying feelings of confidence and self-esteem. To this day, whenever Steven feels anxious about a situation, he fires his anchor and is able to recreate the positive feelings evoked by his 'action stations' DVD.

Visualisation can also help us to overcome negative memories, especially if we have a particularly unhappy DVD that overwhelms us and stops us thinking rationally. You will remember that I described one of the ways we try to cope with very powerful negative memories is to place them in quarantine on a high shelf at the back of the mind's library. Despite this, strong negative memories still manage to get through the filter when a trigger causes a flashback. Occasionally, the flashback occurs when we're asleep and we have a nightmare. This makes it difficult to challenge thinking errors in the normal way.

My client Chlöe, a social worker, was involved in a road rage incident. A blue BMW swerved in front of her car, causing her to brake heavily. The BMW's driver got out of his car, shouted at Chlöe, smashed her car's windscreen and drove off. After the incident, every time Chlöe saw a blue BMW she got a flashback of the road rage and became very anxious and panicky. To dilute the strong feelings this powerful negative memory evoked, Chlöe needed to replay the DVD in a controlled way. By dealing with the negative memory, she was able to file DVD on an appropriate shelf, knowing that it no longer had the power to cause her to panic. Having confronted the memory, she was able to come to terms with it as a part of her life experience. Chlöe used a very positive memory of the day she was awarded her post-graduate diploma as a contrast to the negative one. This DVD had a positive effect on Chlöe, making her feel calm and confident when she recalled the diploma ceremony at which her husband and parents had watched her getting her award.

Are there any sad or unhappy DVDs that you feel you need to work on?

- ....
- ....
- ....
- ....

To use the visualisation technique for diluting negative memories, you need two DVDs: the negative memory that's causing the problem and a very positive memory. The positive memory should preferably be one that generates the opposite feeling to the negative. For example, if the negative memory is full of sadness, powerlessness or anxiety, the positive one should be full of happiness, empowerment or confidence. Using this technique involves taking the negative memory and deliberately changing what you see, hear and feel, as if you were editing a DVD and showing it on a television screen, practising controlling the negative memory and its power to cause negative feelings. Then, like Chlöe in the example above, linking the negative memory to the positive memory, enhancing it to make the positive memory even stronger. Eventually, linking the two memories in this order makes the negative memory the trigger for the positive one. Don't worry if the negative memory makes you feel very anxious to begin with. The anxiety soon reduces as you confront the negative DVD and get used to the emotions.

Take your negative DVD and begin to watch it with your
eyes closed. Imagine that you're watching it on a television for
which you have a special 'remote control'. You're going to dis-
sociate yourself from the memory, so that when you appear in
the DVD, you're watching yourself on the television, from a
distance. As you watch the DVD, note the different colours that
are there and use the remote control to reduce them to black
and white. Once you've changed it into a black and white film,
use the remote control to turn the sound all the way down until
it's become silent. Watch the people in the film opening and
closing their mouths, without any sound coming out. The DVD
looks like an old-fashioned, black and white, silent film from
years ago. Then turn the film into slow motion, so the charac-
ters' movements become surreal. Now adjust the contrast, so
that the quality of the picture becomes very poor and it looks
like there's a snowstorm on the screen. Notice how the images
become more blurred. Finally, press the button on the remote
control that shrinks the film down to a white dot in the centre
of the screen. Click and drag this dot to the top left corner of
the screen, then press another button on the remote control.
Now, the screen becomes filled by a very positive DVD.

As you watch the images in this DVD, notice the colours;
adjust them so they are as bright and vivid as possible. You're
going to associate yourself with this DVD, so that when you
appear, you don't see yourself as a character, you are the person
in the film. The view on the screen is seen through your eyes.
Enjoy looking at the rich colours and then tune the sound, so
that it's wonderfully clear without being loud. Make the sound
stereo; perhaps play your favourite music as a soundtrack to
accompany the pictures. You can see all the detail on the faces
of the people in this positive DVD and hear their voices clearly.
Adjust the temperature in the scene, using the remote control,

so that it's really comfortable, neither too hot nor too cool. Make the pictures as sharp as possible by adjusting the contrast. Finally, at the most positive point in the film, freeze the frame and admire the picture you've just created in wonderful technicolor and listen to the beautiful soundtrack.

Now 'anchor' this positive picture to two things: first, anchor the picture to a word or phrase that you associate with the positive memory and second to an unobtrusive but unusual gesture (a gesture that you only associate with the anchor). Look at the picture, concentrate hard on it and say the word out loud while making the gesture, connecting the anchor to the positive feelings you have when you look at the picture and listen to the soundtrack. Then press the button on the remote control and shrink the picture down to a dot. Click and drag the dot to the bottom right corner of the screen.

Now go to the 'negative' dot in the top left of the screen and drag it to the centre, open the negative dot and run the DVD. Repeat the process of dissociating from the negative memory: make the DVD black and white, silent and in slow motion, create the snowstorm, shrink it to the dot and drag it back to the top left corner of the screen. Then go to the bottom right and use the remote control to drag the positive dot to the centre of the screen and run the DVD. Repeat the process of associating with the positive memory: enhance the colours, give it a soundtrack, adjust the temperature, sharpen the images, freeze the frame and anchor the picture, soundtrack and positive feelings to your chosen phrase or word and the physical gesture. Shrink the picture down and drag it to the bottom right corner of the screen. Repeat the same process once more with each DVD.

Negative memories sometimes pop into our heads for no apparent reason, particularly if they're triggered subconsciously, as when Maureen eventually recognised that the smell of floor polish operated as the subconscious trigger for the negative DVDs of her previous job. Subconscious triggers can make it difficult to prevent a negative memory from coming into our minds. However, by practising the visualisation technique we can use the negative DVD as the cue to trigger the positive, by connecting the two closely. It's important to run the DVDs in the same order: first the negative DVD, then the positive. This ensures that the positive memory doesn't become the trigger for the negative one.

Visualisation is also a very useful technique for dealing with nervousness and anxiety. It works well as a relaxation technique and can be very useful in helping people to sleep. And visualisation has been very successful outside the clinical field, especially in sports psychology. For many years I worked for the National Coaching Foundation and delivered training programmes to help sports coaches use visualisation. Visualisation has been used in sport in different ways: to help athletes relax, to promote feelings of self-confidence and, by visualising future events, to increase the likelihood of positive self-fulfilling prophecies. Johnny Wilkinson, the England rugby player, used visualisation every time he took a penalty kick. By visualising what a successful penalty kick would look, sound and feel like, Wilkinson programmed his mind so that his body delivered the successful outcome. Visit our website (www.mindhealthdevelopment. co.uk) for more information and free relaxation downloads which can help problems such as anxiety and sleeplessness.

Summary of Step 4

This step has focused on techniques and exercises to help you to use your positive mind to make you happier and more confident. The more you add to your positive list, the more diary entries you complete, the more Plus 4s you engage in and the more often you express your gratitude, the more successful you'll be in systematically challenging your thinking errors. Visualisation can be used when you want to enhance a positive DVD to help you relax or feel more confident. If you have a particularly unhappy memory that's preventing you challenging thinking errors in the normal way, visualisation can help by diluting the memory and linking it to a positive one.

After a little practice in these various techniques, you'll start to notice the improvements in your thinking. Don't give up too easily: it won't happen immediately but with effort, you'll soon find that you're feeling happier about your life. Different techniques work for different people, so try them all and use the ones that work for you.

Practice makes permanent

For positive thinking to become habitual we have to practice constantly challenging our thinking errors.

Well-formed outcomes

By answering the seven questions to establish our WFOs, we can clearly see what we want and the changes we need to make.

The positive list

Completing a positive list is a simple way to practice challenging thinking errors and re-set our filter.

Keeping a diary

Using a diary helps us to systematically challenge thinking errors every day.

Plus 4s

The scores in the diary tend to be higher if we do a Plus 4 activity each day. And the distraction of doing Plus 4s helps take our mind off our troubles.

The gratitude list

Consciously being grateful is a wonderful way to challenge our thinking errors and keep us psychologically healthy.

Visualisation

Visualisation can be used to make a positive memory even better or to dilute the power of a negative memory.

STEP   5

Know what you can control and let go
of what you can't

Broadly speaking, the more control we have in our lives, the more positive DVDs we end up playing. However, sometimes we have to accept that there are certain situations we can't control.

I once taught a post-graduate class for teachers in Ohio, USA. One of the class members was a woman with quite a forceful, dominant personality. When we discussed what made an effective learning environment, she was quite dismissive of others in the group who felt that students should play a part in deciding what that environment should be. As the day grew warmer, the woman removed her sweatshirt; underneath was a tee shirt with the message 'Because I'm the teacher!'

Believing we can control other people's behaviour because of our personality or our position of authority can easily set us up for failure. The only behaviour we can truly control is our own.

Control and stress

In difficult situations, people who feel helpless and unable to control or influence the situation usually suffer higher levels of stress. A study of British civil servants found that the more control they had over their work, the lower the levels of stress they experienced.[23] While this seems a pretty obvious conclusion, the relationship between control and stress may be slightly more complex. Although it seems clear that the more control we have over our lives the less stress we feel, some people who have very little control over a situation can experience relatively low levels of stress if they're able to 'let it go'.

The highest levels of stress seem to occur when someone can neither control a situation fully nor let it go. Accepting that we have relatively little control over certain situations can be very liberating – providing that we then channel our energies into the situations that we can control (see Figure 7). Eleanor came to me in a very depressed state. Her marriage was falling apart, the family had financial problems and she was struggling to cope with her job. However, perhaps her biggest difficulty was that her nine and eleven year old sons constantly disobeyed her. She started crying as she described taking her sons to school one day.

Arriving at the school gates, both boys refused to get out of the car. The eldest eventually decided to get out and walked into school. However her youngest, Phillip, refused to leave the car and stayed in the front passenger seat. In desperation, she got out of the car and walked round to the front passenger

Control Levels and Stress Levels

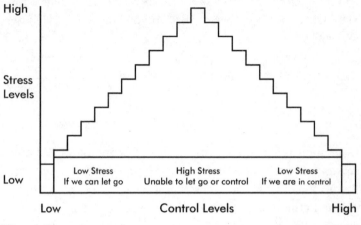

Figure 7

door, so she could physically march him into school. As she approached the door, Phillip jumped across to the driver's seat and hid down by the pedals where his mum couldn't reach him. As Eleanor ran round to the driver's door Phillip jumped back to the other seat and hid on the floor where again she could not reach him. This game of cat and mouse continued for several minutes, with Eleanor becoming more and more stressed, much to the bemusement of the other parents dropping their children off. Eventually, she managed to catch hold of Phillip's arm and dragged him out of the car. As she marched him across the playground, Phillip threw himself on the ground and began to shout and scream. Eleanor's humiliation was complete when one of the teachers told Phillip to get up immediately, stop shouting and go into school, which he did straight away.

As Eleanor told me this story the tears rolled down her face. Her inability to control Phillip's behaviour had been seen by parents and teachers, some of whom spoke disparagingly about Eleanor's parenting skills. Eleanor said she felt like a complete failure. 'Whose behaviour can you control?' I asked her. She paused for a long time and replied: 'Only my own.' It's hard for many parents to accept that their children have minds of their own and won't automatically do as they ask.

Choices and consequences

Listening to Eleanor, it became clear that she often had arguments with both her sons. She had become very threat sensitive, due to the difficult life events she was experiencing; when she got up in the morning her filters were set to notice every little negative thing about her life in general and the children's behaviour in particular. She constantly challenged them about their behaviour, which provoked rows during which Eleanor often lost her temper and shouted at the boys. Her increased anxiety levels affected her confidence in her ability to get the children to behave. The boys sensed Eleanor's lack of confidence and were more aggressive in challenging her authority; a negative self-fulfilling prophecy.

I suggested a fairly simple plan, based on the theory of choices and consequences, to help Eleanor.[24] First, Eleanor had to accept that she couldn't control the children's behaviour; she could only control her own. This meant that, despite the boys' outbursts, Eleanor would control her temper and not shout at them. Second, I asked Eleanor to work out which two or three aspects of their behaviour were completely unacceptable. One was, not surprisingly, the refusal to go to school. These were to be our 'hills worth dying for'; the rest of their behaviour we called 'background noise', not worth getting into an argument about. Eleanor would just let these issues go. Next, Eleanor

would make it absolutely clear to the children that if they chose
to ignore her on the 'hill' issues there would be negative consequences. If they chose to work with her on the hill issues there
would be positive consequences. If Eleanor recognised that the
children were making 'background noise', minor bad behaviour, she would ignore the behaviour and let it go. She would
save her energy and stop getting drawn into the background
noise, so that she could rechannel that energy into dealing with
the hills.

When we first talked, Eleanor seemed a little uneasy about
simply ignoring some of the boys' minor bad behaviours. I asked
her: 'In terms of changing their behaviour, how effective is
your current strategy of challenging them on every issue?' She
paused, smiled ruefully and admitted it hadn't worked. I pointed
out it was quite possible that, to begin with, our plan to change
their behaviour wouldn't work either but at least by controlling
her behaviour she'd feel better about not shouting and wouldn't
have the stress and anxiety of the rows. Eleanor seemed much
happier but still had one problem with the plan: 'If I just ignore
their minor bad behaviour it will look like I think it's okay.' We
agreed it was legitimate for Eleanor to tell her children that she
was disappointed with them if they behaved badly in small ways
but she would simply make the statement and not get into an
argument.

Eventually, Eleanor began to accept that she couldn't completely control her children's behaviour. However, as long as
she controlled her behaviour, she felt calmer and more in control of the situation. When she felt calm Eleanor was able to
explain to the children that it was their decision about how to
behave on the 'hill' issues but if they chose to ignore her, there
would be consequences. This example shows how accepting
that we can't control some things allows us to save our energy

and put it into what we can control. Eleanor accepted she couldn't directly control Phillip's behaviour but by remaining calm, not losing her temper or shouting at Phillip, she felt more positive about herself and therefore more able to deal with the situation.

The next time Phillip began to play the game of refusing to get out of the car, Eleanor's plan worked very effectively. She had explained her problem to Phillip's teacher and warned her that although Phillip might be late for school, she needed the teacher's support. Phillip's teacher was happy to provide this support when she understood Eleanor's problem. She also reassured Eleanor that there weren't any problems with Phillip in school; he was always happy and well-behaved. Eleanor also warned her boss that she might be a little late getting to work because she was having difficulties with her son, but offered to make the time up later in the day. Once again she got a positive response. This made Eleanor feel confident and in control even before she arrived at school.

When Phillip began the game of jumping from seat to seat, Eleanor got back into the driver's seat and told Phillip calmly that it was his choice whether he continued to play this game but she wasn't prepared to play it with him. She explained why she wanted him to get out of the car and walk into school like the other children and that if he chose not to do so, he would not be allowed to play with his friends after school. Phillip refused to leave the car. Eleanor said she thought it was a shame; it was his choice to ignore her but he knew what the consequence would be. Phillip began to shout and scream that it was unfair. Eleanor calmly picked up her newspaper and started reading it. Eventually Phillip calmed down; when he was calm, Eleanor asked him very politely if he would get out of the car and walk with her into school. After a few minutes, Phillip left the car quietly and Eleanor thanked him as they walked into school together. She also promised him that if he was good about getting out of the car the next day, he would be able to play with his friends.

Eleanor was able to control her own behaviour when dealing with Phillip. She was also able to convince Phillip's teacher and her boss to support her in dealing with Phillip's behaviour. This increased her feelings of control. Regardless of how Phillip behaved, she would have recorded a positive memory of how she successfully controlled her behaviour and got the support of two key people. There were two further benefits: first, if Eleanor had a difficult day in the future and lost her patience with Phillip (almost certain, because she's only human!) she would be able to challenge the thinking error that, 'I *never* seem to be able to deal calmly with Phillip'. She can search her mental DVD library and find the positive memory of herself managing his tantrums effectively, which will disprove the thinking error that she can't deal calmly with him. Second, she's better equipped to break the cycle of negative self-fulfilling prophecies. The confidence she gained from dealing with Phillip calmly in the past will increase her belief that she can successfully do it in the future.

If you're currently dealing with a stressful situation which is causing you anxiety because it involves somebody else's negative behaviour you might find the next exercise useful. This exercise isn't limited to dealing with children; it can be effective in dealing with negative adults in certain situations.

Think about the negative behaviour: what are the 'hills worth dying for'? (Select two or three 'hills')

- ....
- ....
- ....
- ....

What behaviour is just background noise?

- ....
- ....
- ....
- ....

What are the positive consequences for the person if they choose to work with you?

- ....
- ....
- ....
- ....

What are the negative consequences for the person if they choose to work against you?

- ....
- ....
- ....
- ....

Whose support do you need if you're going to be successful contesting the 'hills'?

- ....
- ....
- ....
- ....

- **Tip:** *Don't reinforce bad behaviour, do reinforce good behaviour.* Ignoring minor bad behaviour, especially in children, is usually far more effective than making every issue a hill. However, if the issue is a hill then address it every single time. Be consistent – consistently refuse to be drawn into background noise and consistently tackle the hills by giving the person choices and consequences. Once you've had some success dealing with the hills, reprioritise the behaviour; repeated background noise may become the next hill to climb. When reinforcing good behaviour, you don't have to reward it every time (in fact it's better not to) but it can be very effective to make a point of thanking someone who has behaved well and occasionally reward their good behaviour.

- **Tip:** *Try to understand why the person doesn't want to do what you're asking them.* It's often best to revisit things when everyone has calmed down. By understanding their point of view, you may be able to reach a compromise.
- **Tip**: *Use relaxation exercises to help let go.* There are many good relaxation exercises to help people feeling very stressed to unwind. When we are in a relaxed state of mind we are more susceptible to changing our perception so that we can let go of the things we can't control.

Getting a balanced view

Understanding the balance between what we can control and where we have very little control is vital for good psychological health. Making excuses and blaming other people when we could have controlled a situation disempowers us. Blaming ourselves when we really couldn't have controlled a situation leads to the thinking error of personalisation – seeing ourselves as being responsible for a negative event over which we had no control.

We need to find the balance between disempowerment and personalisation. People who disempower themselves need to recognise that with more determination they could control some situations. Individuals who make the error of personalisation need to recognise they can't control every situation (see Figure 8).

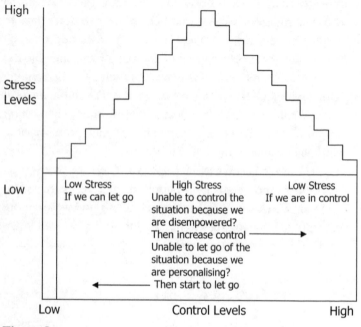

Figure 8

Robyn was a woman in her early forties who had gone through a bitter divorce from her husband Nick. Nick was very volatile and unpredictable and sometimes drank heavily. During their marriage he had often been verbally abusive towards Robyn and occasionally used threats, intimidation and minor violence. Nick and Robyn had two children; because of Nick's unwillingness to compromise, a complicated legal schedule of parental rights for weekend and holiday arrangements for the children had been drawn up.

Robyn became very stressed and anxious every time an unexpected change looked as if it would affect the schedule.

If she contacted Nick to explain, she usually got an angry email threatening her with court action if she did not stick to the letter of the schedule. On one occasion, Robyn booked a foreign holiday during the children's summer break. She was due to hand the children over to Nick on the day after they returned from holiday. Unfortunately, the tour operator changed the flight times at short notice, meaning she wouldn't be able to hand the children over to Nick on schedule. As Robyn talked, she was completely resigned to cancelling the holiday and losing a lot of money. I asked her if she could speak to Nick, to see if he could be flexible. She told me she'd tried but had received an email threatening that if she did not hand the children over at the original time he would take her to court.

Robyn shrugged her shoulders and said there was nothing she could do. I asked her to consider all her possible options. She described a number of options, including going to court and fighting Nick. I asked her what was stopping her from doing that. Robyn told me that she didn't want the cost of a legal battle. She'd had such a horrible time in court over the divorce that she didn't think she could go through it again and 'anyway he'd probably win he always does'. Robyn was disempowering herself by making negative assumptions: it would cost a lot of money to take legal advice, it would definitely go to court, it would be as unpleasant as the original court case and she would lose the case anyway. I asked Robyn if she knew any lawyers who might be able to give her an opinion without too much expense. She thought for a while and remembered that one of her friends had a son, Tony, who was a lawyer. She paused; she was sure Tony would have a chat with her and give her some advice. She agreed to meet her friend and Tony before our next session.

The next time I saw Robyn, she was much more positive. Tony had been very helpful, offering to write a letter to Nick's solicitor on Robyn's behalf. He thought that if Nick did take Robyn to court over access, there was a strong likelihood the court would find in Robyn's favour and anyway, the costs would be quite modest. Tony also made an interesting point – it was possible it might go to court, and she could lose, but at least she'd feel she'd stood up to Nick. In the end, Nick backed down and agreed to the children being handed over after they had returned from their holiday. If Robyn had disempowered herself she would have missed out on a holiday, lost quite a lot of money and continued to be intimidated by Nick. As Robyn said to me at our last session: 'I think I spent so long being intimidated by Nick, both throughout our marriage and since we've been divorced, that every time he threatened me with court I just rolled over and gave in. Having stood up to him once I know I could do it again ... and now Nick knows that too.'

This example demonstrates the balance needed over control. The problem lay partly in the difficulty of the situation and partly with Robyn's behaviour: Nick had intimidated Robyn for years but her unwillingness to take control left her disempowered. The next story is an example of someone trying too hard to take control, resulting in personalisation.

Adrian was a senior hospital administrator. He had become increasingly anxious at the many changes to the National Health Service, which were directly affecting his hospital. The changes, which were driven by the government, had resulted in low morale among the hospital's staff, for which Adrian felt personally responsible. Adrian had no choice but to implement the changes, regardless of whether he agreed with them or not. He spent an increasing amount of time trying to find ways to avoid implementing the changes or to implement them in ways that might affect his hospital less but he was fighting a losing battle.

Adrian believed that his inability to hold back change and the staff's resulting low morale were his personal failures. He was making the thinking error of personalisation. No hospital administrator in the country could have made any difference to the changes that the government wanted. As Adrian began to see this, he started to work on issues he could control, such as reducing waiting lists for surgery within his hospital. Not surprisingly, he began to feel much better about himself and less stressed about accepting that there were some issues he had to let go.

The study of prisoners offers an interesting perspective on how to combine a balanced view on control. In most respects, prisoners have very little control over their lives, because their freedom has been taken from them. My colleague Glyn often tells the uplifting story of Victor Frankl, an Austrian Jew imprisoned by the Nazis in the brutal Auschwitz concentration camp.[25] The concentration camp's daily routine consisted of terrible physical and mental tortures. Prisoners were slowly starved to death, in appalling conditions, under the constant threat of the gas chambers. Frankl had seen several members of his family taken to the gas chambers and murdered. It would have been very understandable if he had completely given up hope, as so many of his fellow prisoners did.

Before his imprisonment Frankl had been a university professor. While he was imprisoned, he wondered what, if he survived, he would teach his students about his experiences in Auschwitz. He realised that if he wanted to be able to tell a positive story about his experiences, he had to live those positive experiences in the here and now. He set about creating a series of positive memories that he could use in the future. The only things he could control were his attitude and behaviour, so he became as supportive as he possibly could to his fellow prisoners, talking to them, sympathising with them, showing them every kindness he could. He became a wonderful source of inspiration, not only for the other prisoners but also for some of the guards. Like Admiral Stockdale, Frankl was planning for the day he would be released; balancing the brutal truth with an optimism born of trying to control as much of his life as possible by creating positive memories that he could use in the future. Frankl said: 'Everything can be taken away from us but one thing, the last human freedom, to choose one's own attitude in any given set of circumstances, to choose our own way.'

Think of a situation that's causing you some stress or anxiety. What have you already done to try to control it?

- ....
- ....
- ....
- ....

What can you actually control? (What talents, knowledge and experience can you use to help control the situation? How can you be more influential?)

- ....
- ....
- ....
- ....

What do you need to let go? (What factors do other people control?)

- ....
- ....
- ....
- ....

How can you try to change your perception of the situation or other people? (Which negative emotions can you change?)

- ....
- ....
- ....
- ....
- **Tip:** *Check out your perception with other people.* When the lack of control is real there may not be much we can do to directly affect the situation. Where the lack of control is perceived, it's important to generate a number of available options, think through them and reflect on them. Use friends or family to help you check out your perception and generate options; you may be more in control than you think.
- **Tip:** *Redefine success.* Instead of defining success in terms of what you can't control, define success in terms of what you can control. Success for Robyn wasn't winning a court case – which would have been up to the judge – success was standing up to Nick, which was in Robyn's control.
- **Tip:** *Write down everything you've done to try to control the situation.* It's easier to let go if you feel you've already done everything you can.

Imagine the nightmare comes true

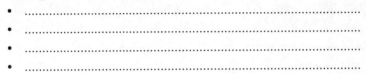

Sometimes we're faced with a very serious and worrying situation over which we have little control. In these circumstances we might need to consider facing up to the brutal truth.

I counselled a surgeon, Marcia, who was under investigation for malpractice. Marcia had completed an operation using a laser, which had malfunctioned and burned her patient, who was now suing Marcia. Marcia was so anxious about making another mistake while operating that she was in danger of falling into the trap of self-fulfilling prophecy. I asked Marcia to think about the worst case scenario: 'Imagine the nightmare comes true and write a plan for dealing with it.' When she came back, she told me:

> The worst case scenario is that I could be struck off the medical register. I wouldn't go to prison, because the worst the investigators could prove was negligence, not deliberate recklessness. If I got struck off we wouldn't starve; my husband is a teacher and although he earns less than me, we could still pay most of our bills if we reduced our expenditure. I would then go back to college and study law. I enjoyed studying when I did my medical degree and I've always had an interest in law. I know it would take a few years but if I qualified as a lawyer I would specialise in legal cases of medical negligence … and with my background I think I'd be pretty good at it!

If, like Marcia, you're facing a very serious and worrying situation, try this exercise:

What's the worst thing that could happen?

- ....
- ....
- ....
- ....

What would the consequences be?

- ....
- ....
- ....
- ....

What would your options be for dealing with the consequences?

- ....
- ....
- ....
- ....

What similar situations have you experienced that might help
you deal with the consequences?

- ....
- ....
- ....
- ....

Whose help or support could you call on?

- ....
- ....
- ....
- ....

- **Tip:** *Think about the story you want to tell when it's over.*
  Take a leaf out of Frankl's book: when this challenging situation is over, think about how you would like to be able
  to describe the way you behaved and start behaving that
  way now.

The power of forgiveness

Earlier, I mentioned that people who focus on situations over
which they have no control often end up blaming or accusing
other people, thereby disempowering themselves and increasing their feelings of victimisation. But how do we let go in
situations where other people genuinely are to blame for some
of our problems? One way is to use the power of forgiveness.

Some years ago, I counselled an electrician, Colin, who was in his early thirties. When he was a teenager, Colin's mother had left his father to start a new relationship. Colin continued to live with his father, with whom he got on very well but when Colin was seventeen, his father met another woman, Sonia. Very soon, Colin's father decided to marry Sonia, who moved into the family home with her young daughter. Colin and Sonia had a very poor relationship; they often argued and had rows. Eventually, his father told Colin to leave. The experience of his mother leaving and his father 'throwing him out' left Colin very prone to stress, anxiety and depression. Perhaps justifiably, he blamed his father for his psychological health problems. As Colin recalled his experiences, he remained very bitter about what his father had done fifteen years before. Since that time, he had refused to speak to his father, even when they had recently met at a family wedding. Colin remarked that he often drove past his father's house and whenever he did, he started playing the negative DVDs of the time his father told him to leave home.

I could see the painful DVD playing in Colin's mind as he said, 'I'll never forgive my dad for what he did to me.' Colin was still a victim of what his father had done many years before. I asked Colin who he was punishing by not forgiving his father: 'My dad of course, it's his loss that he'll never speak to me again.' I asked him who else was suffering through this behaviour. Colin was silent for a while and then said: 'Me. I don't suppose my dad is even aware of what I'm feeling when I drive past his house and think of what he did to me when I was just seventeen.'

Colin and I spent some time talking about what had happened and eventually Colin came to see that he was partly to blame for the rows with Sonia. He also saw that his father was frightened Sonia might walk out if he didn't tell Colin to leave home. Perhaps most important, Colin recognised that by not forgiving his father he continued to be a victim of an act that had taken place many years before. Colin summarised this at the end of the counselling:

> I can't forget what happened to me, the DVD memories are there at the back of the library and every time I pass the house they start playing. But I think I've learned to let go of the pain and anger by focusing on some of the positive DVD memories I have of my dad and by realising that he was only human. He was obviously hurt when my mum left him and he was scared of losing his second wife. I can understand what he did but I don't necessarily agree with him. I'm not ready for reconciliation just yet but in time I think this could happen because I don't feel like a victim any more.

Holding on to the anger and bitterness we feel towards another person is like drinking poison and expecting the other person to die. But sometimes blaming ourselves can be just as damaging. Anxiety disorders and depression are often brought on by guilt, which is the result of self-blame. A client of mine, Harry, felt very sad and guilty over his mother's death in a nursing home. At the inquest into her death, the coroner noted that the staff of the nursing home hadn't lived up to their duty of care towards his mum; something Harry hadn't noticed. The guilt was worsened because Harry was a qualified nurse and believed he should have been aware of the home's lack of care. ('Should' statements are one of the nine thinking errors.)

Harry felt very guilty and very remorseful of his own failings. Fortunately, through the counselling, he was able to change his perceptions. He recognised that because he was a nurse, his father and two sisters had allowed Harry to liaise with the staff at the nursing home. Harry's father, in particular, had not wanted to deal with the medical issues. Harry had tried to be optimistic for his father and sisters by emphasising the positive elements of his mother's treatment and consequently hadn't noticed the lack of care in certain areas. Harry had also forgotten that he was only human; although he was a qualified nurse, he was also an anxious son who was worried about the health of his mother: in that situation, most people would be unable to think as clearly as usual. Harry couldn't review his mum's treatment plan in the same professional and objective way he could view the treatment plan of one of his own patients. Eventually, Harry was able to forgive himself by challenging the 'should statements' holding the filter in place so only the negative DVDs of his mother's last days played.

Colin and Harry are good examples of people who were able to change their perception of something that happened in the past. Because we can't control the past, we have to try to learn from it and let go. Colin and Harry were able to forgive and let go of the negative emotions that they experienced every time they replayed the painful DVDs.

Think of a situation in which you feel someone was to blame for something: who needs forgiveness?

- ....
- ....
- ....
- ....

What needs to be forgiven?

- ....
- ....
- ....
- ....

What other pressures may have caused this person to do what they've done?

- ....
- ....
- ....
- ....

How are you suffering now by not forgiving this person?

- ....
- ....
- ....
- ....

What are the positive traits of this person?

- ....
- ....
- ....
- ....

What could be done to help reconcile the situation?

- ....
- ....
- ....
- ....

What have you learned from this experience?

- ....
- ....
- ....
- ....

- **Tip:** *Remember Fundamental Attribution Errors.* This is the basic mistake we make of attributing the blame to the person and forgetting to take into account the pressure of the situation. I mentioned the example of Marcus Aurelius taking into account people's situations in explaining their behaviour – people often act in a negative way if they are under extreme pressure.

- **Tip:** *Let he who has not sinned cast the first stone.* Think of a time when you did something you now regret; hopefully someone forgave you. None of us are saints, we all make mistakes.

Solution fixation

We've established that letting go of what we really can't control and channelling our energies into what we can control gives us greater balance but why do we find it so hard to let go sometimes? One of the reasons is that we can become almost obsessed with trying to solve a problem. My colleague Glyn has created a name for this concept: solution fixation. We become fixated on trying to find a solution for a problem that can't be solved. The fixation increases our anxiety and because the problem can't be solved, this reinforces the idea that we're a failure.

Lesley had been anxious for many years. The roots of her anxiety reached back to her childhood: she had never known her father and her mother had died when she was twelve years old, after which she and her younger sister were brought up in care. After working with me for a few weeks Lesley began to understand herself better; however, she still got very frustrated with her anxiety. She mentioned one day that she'd invited a friend to her house for dinner at the weekend: 'I don't know why I always get so anxious when friends arrive at the house but it only lasts until they've been with me for about fifteen minutes, then it goes.' It became clear as we talked that Lesley's anxiety wasn't specific to this particular friend or this particular occasion: she was often anxious when people visited her home.

'It's really silly, I've already started to worry about the weekend and it's only Monday today! I'll end up spending hours trying to think about what I can do to stop the fifteen minutes of anxiety.' Lesley spent so much time fixating on trying to solve her anxiety that the solution fixation was causing her more stress than the anxiety itself.

Lesley learned to recognise that her anxiety was a deep-rooted consequence of her difficult childhood. The anxiety had become a fairly fixed aspect of her internal make-up. As a result of this insight Lesley was able to accept the anxiety for what it was – fifteen minutes of moderate discomfort that wasn't worth hours of worry trying to solve. Letting go of solution-fixation significantly reduced Lesley's overall anxiety levels.

Is there an aspect of your personality you don't like, which if you learned to accept rather than try to change would save you a lot of worry?

Summary of Step 5

In this step, we've focused on knowing what we can control and letting go of what we can't. Occasionally, we fall into the trap of disempowering ourselves and we give up too easily when, with a little more determination, we might succeed in controlling the outcome. In some situations, we blame ourselves for things going wrong when we couldn't have controlled the outcome. As the song says, 'You can plan a pretty picnic but you can't control the weather'.

Knowing what we can control and letting go of what we can't helps us to use our energy more productively. If we're using our energy productively we'll create more positive than negative DVDs, which will make us feel better about our world and ourselves.

Control and stress

The more control we have over a situation the less stress or anxiety we experience. But it's possible to have low levels of control and low levels of stress if we can let go of the things we can't control.

Choices and consequences

It's important to accept that people have choices about how they behave and that all we can do is to try to influence their choices through controlling our behaviour.

Imagine the nightmare comes true

Facing up to the worst case scenario and writing a plan to deal with it helps us to recognise that we have more control over a situation than we believe.

Getting a balanced perspective on control

Making the effort to control what we can empowers us. When we disempower ourselves we make excuses and blame other people. However, we need a balance: failing to recognise there are some situations we can't control leads to an irrational sense of failure.

The power of forgiveness

Being able to forgive others or ourselves helps lessen our feelings of bitterness or guilt.

Solution fixation

Many people become so fixated with trying to solve a problem that they lose sight of the fact that it might be impossible to solve.

S T E P 6

Learn how to move forward

When many of my clients first come to see me they often say, 'I just want to go back to being the old me.' After they've mastered the techniques I've covered so far, they start to realise that instead of going back, they need to move forward to develop and grow. But moving forward requires a different kind of thinking. We have to start taking a few risks.

Risk – the currency of the gods

Most people suffering from psychological health problems have acquired the habits of unhappiness: threat sensitivity, pessimism and risk aversion. In business, it's said that risk is the currency of the gods, because it can lead to great wealth. However, risk is the natural enemy of threat sensitive people, who don't take opportunities when there's an element of change or uncertainty. Moving forward means learning to be more optimistic, so that you can take some simple risks. I'm not referring risks that put you in danger but adopting behaviours that take you just out of your comfort zone and help you grow as a person.

The importance of play

Stress and depression have two aspects: negative thinking patterns and lack of participation in activities, especially activities we enjoy. It's easy to see how the two combine to lead people into a negative cycle. When the conscious mind is filtered a steady diet of negative DVDs, the consequent anxiety, self-doubt and lack of confidence mean we often stop engaging in activities that give us pleasure. Re-establishing some of these behaviours is a simple step to moving forward.

As you begin to think more positively, take up an activity that you enjoy. Participating in an enjoyable activity switches on the parasympathetic nervous system and floods the brain with neurotransmitters, such as serotonin, which make you feel good. It can be any activity as long as it's fun, enjoyable or gives you a sense of achievement. Plenty of research, including some of mine, suggests that sport and exercise are particularly helpful in combating stress; however, there's no point taking up anything you don't enjoy.[26] My clients have chosen activities such as gardening, playing the piano, dancing, horse riding, reading, swimming, walking, fishing and painting as their 'homework' to help them move forward.

Sometimes people are reluctant to take up an activity, often because of an aversion to a perceived risk. Eleanor told me how she used to go to the gym at least three or four times a week before she became depressed. However, when struggling to cope with her sons' behaviour, she started to lose her confidence. She stopped going to her aerobics classes because she was worried she wouldn't be able to concentrate on following the moves correctly; she was scared she'd look stupid. One of the main reasons she enjoyed the gym previously was that it kept her in good physical shape but since she'd stopped going she'd put on quite a lot of weight.

Even though I'd helped Eleanor to break the cycle of negative thinking, the thought of restarting the aerobics classes made her threat sensitive again. 'What if I can't remember the moves? What if I make a fool of myself? What will people think of me now that I've put on lots of weight?' Persuading Eleanor to grasp an opportunity to do something that she previously enjoyed involved helping her to overcome her threat sensitivity, pessimism and risk aversion. One of the things that helped Eleanor to overcome her aversion to the risk of looking foolish was the old saying I quoted to her when she started raising objections: 'we wouldn't worry about what other people think about us if we realised how rarely they do'. If Eleanor made a mistake in the class or if someone noticed she'd put on weight, it would only be a fleeting thought; we aren't the centre of other people's universes! When you decide to take up an activity that you enjoy, focus on your behaviour, rather than worrying about how other people might react.

Brainstorm some activities that you'd like to start again or something new you've always wanted to try.

- ....
- ....
- ....
- ....

Where can you find out about these activities?

- ....
- ....
- ....
- ....

Who could help you find the time to do this or who might come along and give you some support?

- ....
- ....
- ....
- ....

- **Tip:** *Just do it for ten minutes or try it just once.* Define success as trying an activity for ten minutes or just doing it once. Have a go at something. If you don't enjoy it or if you find you have no talent for it, no problem, you'll still be successful because you tried it. If it doesn't work out there'll be lots of other things on your list that you can do instead.

Proper selfishness

Finding the time to do an activity that we really enjoy is 'proper selfishness' but many people struggle with the idea of putting themselves first to do something they enjoy. An example of proper selfishness is the safety talk given by cabin crew to passengers on an aeroplane flight: 'If the cabin pressure drops, oxygen masks will be released from the overhead compartment. If you're travelling with someone who needs looking after, put your mask on first so that you'll be able to look after the person in your care.'

In the context of everyday life, proper selfishness means that if we sometimes put ourselves first so we can recharge our batteries, others will benefit from our positive energy.[27]

If occasionally finding the time to put themselves first is good for people with anxiety or depression, why do they find it so difficult? The answer lies in the misplaced guilt that comes from the thinking error of 'should statements'. Many people feel that instead of taking part in activities they enjoy they should be doing other things, such as working or caring for their family.

Jessica was a single parent who had been struggling with depression for several months before she started working with me. She'd made great progress and as we began to talk about the importance of play, she recalled how, many years ago, she used to enjoy horse riding. I asked her why she didn't take it up again. She gave me a list of reasons ranging from the cost to not having enough time. But the real reasons were rooted in putting other people first. Her time was filled by her job, looking after her two teenaged children, keeping up with the chores around the house and helping her elderly father. After we discussed the concept of proper selfishness, Jessica eventually agreed to go horse riding as her homework.

When Jessica came to her next session she told me how she'd got up on Saturday morning and told the children that she was going riding for a couple of hours. Driving to the riding school she felt *very* guilty that she was spending time on herself when she should have been doing household chores, shopping for her father or sharing time with her children. But she remembered our discussion on proper selfishness and was able to relax and enjoy her ride. When she got home she noticed she felt much less resentful about doing the chores and looking after the children and her dad, and she had much more energy. Putting herself first and going riding had recharged Jessica's energy, increased her confidence and improved her self-esteem.

Another example of the misplaced guilt that makes some people reluctant to apply proper selfishness is if they've been away from work with stress, anxiety or depression. They feel they shouldn't be doing things they enjoy, because taking part in pleasurable activities seems to be wrong when they're away from work with a psychological illness. The opposite is true; taking part in pleasurable activities is a therapy that will help get them psychologically fit so they can return to work.

Tom was recovering from acute anxiety and panic attacks which had kept him away from work for several weeks. I knew Tom was a keen cyclist and as he got better, I suggested he started riding his bike again. At first he was pleased but then I saw the anxiety start to rise. 'What if someone from work sees me on my bike and they tell my boss?' We agreed that I would call Tom's boss and explain he was making good progress and that riding his bike was part of the therapy to help him make a full recovery. Tom started riding his bike and within two weeks was ready to begin work again.

If you're still reluctant to find the time to put yourself first to do something you enjoy, what or who is stopping you?

- ....
- ....
- ....
- ....

If you applied proper selfishness who would benefit from you recharging your batteries and how would they benefit?

- ....
- ....
- ....
- ....

What are the positive consequences of doing it? What are the negative consequences of not doing it?

- ....
- ....
- ....
- ....

Planning for the future

Successfully applying proper selfishness to do things we enjoy is a clear indication that we're moving forward. But to keep the momentum we have to start thinking about the future. The best way to do this is to begin making plans. Leaving things to chance or spontaneously grasping opportunities as they arise is more difficult if you're prone to threat sensitivity.

Spontaneity requires us to make decisions quickly, which seems much more risky than planning well ahead. By planning ahead, we reduce the perceived risk and get used to the idea that we're going to do something, so it seems a little less scary. Making plans involves creating positive DVDs about the future, which means we get the pleasure of anticipation, something that is missing from spontaneous decision making. Anticipation is beneficial in countering negative thoughts; a bright picture of the future can help improve our mood when we are trying to cope with difficult times in the present.

My experience of counselling clients, particularly those with depression, is that in the depths of their low mood they feel they don't have anything to look forward to. Their filters don't allow them to notice the positive things in the present so it becomes very difficult for them to imagine that there might be anything positive about the future. Resetting their filter not only allows them to see the positive things in the present, it helps them to create a bright future.

A useful technique is to create a list of things to look forward to. The list can be a mixture of the simple and the exotic: holidays, watching your children play, looking forward to a weekend break, going for a picnic in the country, booking a theatre trip, planning to have friends around for a meal, going to a firework party, saving up for a ride in a hot air balloon, going fishing, taking the children to a theme park, Christmas, birthday celebrations or the thought of any future activity that brings a smile to your face.

List a few things you're looking forward to during the next year.

- ....
- ....
- ....
- ....

- **Tip:** *Shared pleasures*. Ask friends and family what they're looking forward to over the next year – perhaps there'll be occasions you can share with them.
- **Tip:** *Write it up.* Transfer the list to your diary, calendar or planner. The more visible it is and the more often that you see enjoyable future events written down, the more likely you are to benefit from the anticipation.

Making plans for work

Planning a range of things to look forward to socially gives us lots to look forward to but for most of us, work plays a pretty important part in our lives. Because of this, when work isn't going well it can cause stress and anxiety.

How happy are you with your job?

- ....

What are the positive aspects of work?

- ....
- ....
- ....
- ....

What are the negative aspects of work?

- ....
- ....
- ....
- ....

How does your job positively affect the rest of your life?

- ....
- ....
- ....
- ....

How does your job negatively affect the rest of your life?

- ....
- ....
- ....
- ....

There's a lot of evidence that shows work is good for us.[28] Our job ensures social contact, structures the week, gives us a sense of achievement, contrasts with and so helps us to appreciate our relaxation time, feeds our self-esteem when we're praised and of course, pays the bills! It's also a great distraction, because it keeps our mind active, which helps us to stop replaying negative DVDs if we're struggling with troubles outside work. But sometimes it's the job itself that's the cause of our problems:

14% of the working population experience work-related stress at a level that makes them ill.

If you're away from work through illness, regardless of the cause, it's important to try to get back to work within a reasonable time: the longer you leave it the more difficult this becomes. You may already have decided that you want to find another job but being away through illness won't help you in the long term. I often tell clients the story of Declan Murphy, a talented jockey who rode horses in National Hunt races in the 1990s. In one fateful race, the horse he was riding fell after jumping a fence and Declan sustained a serious head injury. The doctors who treated him suggested that even if Declan survived, he might have brain damage. Eventually, after many months, Declan made a miraculous recovery from his injuries. He went back to work and rode one more race, which he won ... and then immediately retired from life as a jockey and went into another aspect of horse racing where he was able to put his experience as a jockey to good use.

The moral of the story is that sometimes it's important to get back to work, even if you decide that ultimately you need to change jobs. The psychological benefit Declan gained from his approach was that he retired from racing on his own terms. He overcame any risk aversion he might have had as a result of his injuries and proved he could ride in races if he wanted but then he chose not to.

Getting back to work within a reasonable time has many benefits but if you've been away from work for more than three or four weeks with stress, anxiety or depression, it's important to rehabilitate yourself properly. Rushing straight back to working forty hours a week might result in another period of time away from work that could be even longer than the first.

If you're dissatisfied with your job, it's worth looking at the following exercise to see if you can improve things. How good is the fit between your values and the values of the organisation you work for? How well does the organisation treat its people?

* ....
* ....
* ....
* ....

How good is the fit between your traits and the traits needed to do your job well? Has the job changed since you first started? How much time do you spend each week doing what you enjoy and what you're really good at?

* ....
* ....
* ....
* ....

Does your style fit well with the management style of the organisation? Do you like your manager's style? If you manage people do they like your management style? Do you get enough support to do your job well?

* ....
* ....
* ....
* ....

What have you done to try to resolve the problems of the negative aspects of your job and the impact they might have on you?

* ....
* ....
* ....
* ....

What more could you do? Are you blaming others when you could do something about things yourself? Are you wasting energy on trying to control things that are beyond you?

- ....
- ....
- ....
- ....

The answers to these questions could help you make a plan for discussing your dissatisfactions with someone at work who might be able to offer some support.

Boat-burning

It's surprising how often a chat with your boss can improve things but sometimes no amount of tweaking can cover up the fact that it's time for a change. The same can be said for relationships: while there's no substitute for communication, occasionally we need to take more radical action. However, the idea of 'burning our boats' to leave a job or a relationship might seem very risky and as we discussed earlier, risk is the natural enemy of threat sensitive people.

The phrase 'burning our boats' comes from Greek and Roman legend. Their generals believed that by commanding their soldiers to burn their boats, the knowledge that there was no possibility of retreating and sailing back home would drive the men to fight much harder. While boat-burning might be a great way to drive forward, how do we develop the confidence to take such drastic and potentially risky action? By planning ahead. Making the decision to burn our boats, even if it's some time away, creates a very different, more positive way of thinking. The more planning and research we do, the less risky burning our boats seems.

I had a client, Stephen, who came to see me suffering from severe anxiety. Stephen worked for Social Services and had been helping an elderly gentleman to find a place in sheltered housing. Stephen, a highly principled man, was very upset when the local authority housing department refused his client a place in the complex. In a moment of madness, angered by the injustice of the decision, Stephen made a false entry on the computer database, to enable his client to get the accommodation he needed. The next day, Stephen regretted his action and corrected the false entry. Unfortunately, it had already been spotted by Stephen's boss, who suspended him from work while the incident was investigated, in preparation for a disciplinary hearing.

Stephen was absolutely devastated at the thought that he might lose his job. After a couple of sessions, it became clear that he didn't enjoy his job as much as he used to. We discussed his career options; Stephen felt that in the long term he needed to look at options for making his job more fulfilling. He mentioned he'd often thought of becoming a teacher but he didn't have the confidence to leave his job. However, he faced the added difficulty that his career options could be affected by the outcome of the disciplinary hearing, from which there were only two possible outcomes: reprimand or dismissal. If Stephen got a reprimand, it wouldn't make much difference to his career whether he continued in his present job or if he left Social Services to become a teacher. But if he was sacked, not only would he lose his job but he'd also have to mention it in his application to become a teacher.

The date of the disciplinary hearing had been set for four weeks ahead, which gave Stephen relatively little time to think about what he should do. He had to decide how much he wanted to pursue a career as a teacher and weigh up the chances of being sacked. If the likelihood of being dismissed was high,

Stephen could take a decision that was completely in his control; he could burn his boats and resign before the disciplinary hearing. When I mentioned this, Stephen looked pretty nervous. I suggested that if burning his boats with Social Services was the right thing to do, it would seem a lot less risky if he planned and researched the way forward first. At the end of the session Stephen told me he'd continue to give his options some more thought.

Over the next few weeks Stephen did a great deal of research. From his local university, he found teacher training took only a year; after an interview there, he was offered a place on a course. From his trade union representative, he took advice about the likely outcome of the disciplinary hearing; she thought his chances of being dismissed were about 50:50. Stephen was really worried about how he would cope financially if he resigned and took up the teacher training place but found an agency which could give him temporary part-time work while he was training. Stephen also researched the possibility of renting out his house and moving in with a friend. The rent would more than cover his mortgage and he could move back to his house when he qualified and got a full-time job as a teacher. At our last session, one week before the disciplinary hearing, Stephen told me he had decided to burn his boats. He was going to resign and follow his plan for pursuing a new career.

Boat-burning isn't about taking reckless risks. Most of the time we don't have to make instantaneous decisions; we usually have some time to plan. Even Stephen had a few weeks before he had to make a decision. By planning, researching, taking advice and thinking his options through, he was able to make a well thought-out decision. Once we've realised that we're going to burn our boats at some point in the future we often start to feel better, even if we have to go back to the same situation for a while.

Lola was a quietly-spoken administrator, referred to me for counselling. She was married to Geoff, a retail manager. The couple had a four-year-old daughter and lived in a lovely house but were considerably in debt. Geoff did very little of the housework and the vast majority of the childcare fell on Lola's shoulders. He also had a drink problem: most evenings, he called in at the pub and spent at least two hours there and when he got home, he often had a bottle of wine with his evening meal. Lola said that they didn't do much together as a couple but when they socialised with friends or work colleagues she worried that Geoff would get drunk, which he often did. During the counselling, Lola admitted that before they got married she knew Geoff drank a lot but didn't realise its extent. She had often asked him to cut down on his drinking but he was never able to do it for more than a few days before going back to his old habits.

As a result, Lola felt depressed. She found it very hard to envisage a happy future with Geoff but the thought of burning her boats and leaving him to find somewhere else to live with their daughter made her very anxious. Lola felt her options were pretty limited. She decided to try one last time with Geoff, to see if he would get some help with his drinking. She would ask him to go for counselling and was prepared to go with him to help their relationship. Just like Eleanor with her sons, Lola gave Geoff choices and consequences. If he chose not to stop drinking, the consequence was that Lola would burn her boats and leave.

Over the next few months, Lola remained positive and tried to support Geoff in confronting his alcoholism but at the same time, she started to build her plan for boat-burning if it became necessary. She worked out a way to pay off her debts and began to look at options for living accommodation and help with childcare if she had to leave. Unfortunately Geoff refused to get any help with his alcoholism and although he tried to cut down his drinking, eventually he went back to his old ways. Lola had to face up to the brutal truth and accept that Geoff was not going to change. With the help of her family, she executed her plan for burning her boats and moved into rented accommodation. She was able to manage her finances so that she could survive on her salary and soon found that life was a lot less stressful without Geoff.

If you're facing some difficult challenges that might need a radical and potentially riskier approach, try this exercise.

What goal do you want to achieve? Aim for precise definition: provide as much detail as possible, creating a positive DVD of what this looks, sounds and feels like.

- ....
- ....
- ....
- ....

By when do you want to achieve it? Give yourself a date. It shouldn't be too soon, because you need time to do sufficient planning and research before you start on your actions, but don't put it off for too long.

- ....

What is your halfway milestone? What do you need to have completed to make sure you are halfway to your goal? How will you measure your progress?

- ....
- ....
- ....
- ....

Quarter milestones: on what date will you be a quarter of the way to your goal? What do you need to have completed by then to make sure you're on track for your halfway milestones? How will you measure your progress?

- ....
- ....
- ....
- ....

What do you need to do this week? In the early days, you might need to do a lot of research. Make a list of people who could help you, find information on the Internet, read books written by people who know this subject. The more knowledge you have the less risky it will seem; the more people you talk to the less lonely it will feel.

- ....
- ....
- ....
- ....

- **Tip:** *Work up to it.* To start with, use the plan for minor life changes and work up to boat-burning. Unless you are in a similar position to Stephen, you probably have more time than you think before you need to think about fundamental changes in your life. Planning for minor life changes may only require a few weeks but it's still important to break the plan down into milestones.
- **Tip:** *Plan your ideal world.* Once you've mastered the concept of planning for minor life changes, think about what you'd like your ideal world to look like in two years' time. Where do you want to be living, what sort of job do you want to be doing, how do you want to spend your spare time?

Think about the personal, professional and financial changes that you'd need to make to get there in two years and make them part of your milestones.

Summary of Step 6

The main focus of this step has been on moving forward, by taking opportunities to grow and develop. Inevitably, grasping opportunities and trying something different involves an element of risk. Sometimes, the risks may not pay off but if you remember to redefine success in terms of *your* behaviour (at least you tried) your life will be richer for the experience and your confidence and self-esteem will continue to grow.

Risk – the currency of the gods

Threat sensitive people are less likely to take risks and grasp opportunities.

The importance of play

Taking opportunities to engage in new activities or activities we've neglected can be a simple way to move forward but may involve overcoming risk aversion.

Proper selfishness

Proper selfishness involves putting yourself first, to recharge your batteries so others can benefit from your positive energy.

Looking to the future

Moving forward involves engaging with the future and planning ahead.

Making plans for work

Generally speaking, work is good for us and provides us with lots of benefits.

Boat-burning

Occasionally, to move forward, we need to take drastic action and burn our boats. Planning ahead reduces the perceived risk of boat-burning.

As we come to the end of the book, a last thought. Please remember what I said in the introduction: the six steps aren't magical. Be patient. If you've suffered from stress, anxiety or depression for months or years, you'll need to practise the steps for a little while before you start to gain the benefits ... but when you do, you will find your life is happier!

What are the three most useful steps you've learned from this book which will help you to Think Yourself Happy?

- ....
- ....
- ....

Summary

I hope that through understanding the simple concepts for overcoming stress, anxiety and depression, you will have learnt the six steps to change your life from within. Before we finish I'll briefly re-cap.

Step One – Recognise that you are not alone

Stress and mild anxiety are normal, even healthy, reactions to the challenges we face in life. Anxiety disorders and depression develop when we spend a disproportionate amount of time thinking negative thoughts. Unfortunately, psychological ill-health has become a modern-day plague on twenty-first century society, with a significant proportion of the population suffering.

Step Two – Understand how your negative mind works

The subconscious mind is the library that contains our DVD memories and the conscious mind is the DVD player. Between the two is a cluster of brain cells that acts as a filter that only allows through DVDs that it deems appropriate. Thinking errors – negative assumptions – keep the filter in place, so that it's primed to notice negative things related to our worries and concerns.

Step Three – Realise why you must accept yourself

Once we reach our mid- to late twenties, our internal psychological make-up – values, traits and styles – doesn't change much. The way we interact with the external world – life events, traumatic events and circumstances – dictates our mood. Certain negative events are difficult for everyone to deal with. Depending on our psychological make-up we find some situations more difficult to deal with than others; those people whose make-up was shaped by early exposure to threat sensitivity will generally find it more difficult to deal with stressful situations.

Step Four – Master the use of your positive mind

The secret to using our positive mind is to habitually challenge thinking errors, so that a balance of positive and negative DVDs gets through the filter. Practice makes permanent!

Step Five – Know what you can control and let go of what you can't

Establishing how to channel our energies into what we can control and letting go of what we can't makes us feel more positive.

(a)

(b)

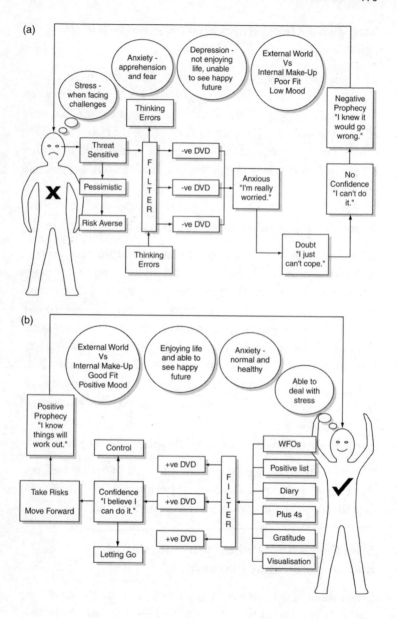

Giving up too easily when we might have been able to exert some influence over a situation disempowers us. However, we can make the thinking error of personalisation if we blame ourselves for failing to hold the tide back when there was really nothing we could have done.

Step Six – Learn how to move forward

Once we've established the habit of thinking more positively in the present, it's time to start to think more positively about the future. However, moving forward involves taking modest risks, which threat sensitive people find quite difficult. We can start taking sensible risks to plan a brighter and more fulfilling future.

Think Yourself Happy!

EPILOGUE ❧

Beach glass

Life is not for the fainthearted. Into every life a little rain must fall. But despite its trials and tribulations, it's still a wonderful life. Nothing demonstrates this better than beach glass.

I was born in the city of Portsmouth and spent many happy hours as a child playing on Southsea beach with my brother, sisters and cousins. Southsea beach is a pebble beach over which, every day, the coastal waters of the English Channel relentlessly roll in on the tides.

As kids, we were interested in the differently shaped pebbles and shells and the various items of flotsam and jetsam washed up by the tide. My treasure from the beach was, and still is, beach glass. Sometimes glass bottles get washed up and the waves smash the bottles against the pebbles. Over the years, the glass is broken into fragments and churned up with the pebbles as the tides roll in and out. The sharp edges of the glass are worn down until they become smooth and the glass is marked by a million scratches, which transform it from a sharp clear shard into a beautiful translucent glass pebble.

I believe this is a metaphor for how we go through life. We start out like that sharp, clear shard of glass, then the tide of life washes us daily against the myriad different pebbles of experience. Over the years, these experiences make their mark upon us, both physically and emotionally. Some of the experiences are happy and joyful, some are sad and painful. We carry the scars and the laughter lines on our bodies and the memories are indelibly etched on our minds.

Each one of us, like every piece of beach glass, is unique and beautiful. The better we are able to see this then the happier and more fulfilled we will be.

Finally, an appeal on behalf of children who may not be able to lead happy and fulfilled lives without some help from us:

Let the Children Live! (www.LetTheChildrenLive.org)

UK Registered Charity No 1013634

PO Box 11

Walsingham

Norfolk

NR22 6EH

UK

They are called 'the disposable ones', the children who live – and sometimes die – in the streets and rubbish dumps of the cities of Colombia in South America. These *gamines*, often unloved, unwanted, beaten, robbed, abused, raped and murdered range in age from six year olds to teenagers.

Although the Colombians are generally a kind and generous people, cocaine traffic-related crime has made cities such as Medellin among the most violent in the world. In the poverty and squalor of the shanty towns, families tend to disintegrate and many children find themselves alone on the street. They have to survive as best they can but they easily fall prey to violence and abuse. Many of the street children sniff glue as an escape from pain, hunger and loneliness.

Let the Children Live is a small registered charity with an enormous and vital task to perform: saving and transforming the lives of as many street children as possible and to prevent other children from having to take to the streets at all. Quite simply, the more funds they can raise, the more children they can reach and the fewer gamines will be disposed of.

A percentage of the profits from the sale of this book is going to support Let the Children Live. However, if everyone who read this book made a contribution to this charity we could make a tremendous difference to the lives of so many children. Please help by making a donation; let's make a difference to the gamines.

Thank you for your kindness.
Rick

Acknowledgements

Writing is a fairly solitary pastime but almost every author receives a lot of help and support from friends and family. I'm no different. A big thank you to:

My dad, who took the time to cast his experienced eye over the boy's work. Your kind comments were much appreciated.

My sister Alexandra, who let me stay in her home in the south of France, where some of this book was written. It's no wonder I didn't want to go home: the food, wine and ambience were very conducive to writing.

My brother Damien, the priest, who said some prayers for the success of the book (well, it would have been silly not to use the family connection).

My sister Josi, who helped me see how difficult life can be for some people, a valuable lesson in writing this book.

My children Sam, Jack and Martha, who were kind enough to be impressed with the old man's efforts.

My friends Sue Wolton, Catherine Thompson and Rosie Riley, who generously gave their time to read and reread the manuscript. Your suggestions were extremely helpful and improved my writing no end.

Juliet Mabey from Oneworld, who never lost faith in the project when others did!

Judith Longman, whose editorial experience proved invaluable and whose patience and encouragement were appreciated.

Ann Grand, whose skilful touch in the final editing of the book made a significant difference.

Glyn Morris, my friend and colleague, for his wise comments, for cave man Dave, for No Permanent Damage, for Solution Fixation and for consistently being great company over a pint or two.

Thanks,
Rick

Mind Health Development

My colleague Glyn Morris and I established Mind Health Development in 2007. It is dedicated to trying to help people to think more positively about their lives, particularly those suffering from stress, anxiety and depression. We work with people and organisations to try to help make a positive contribution to mental health through our cognitive behavioural approach.

Our website (www.mindhealthdevelopment.co.uk) hosts a range of ideas, lots of free information and advice. We offer courses and workshops to people interested in using the cognitive behavioural approach outlined in this book and training for counsellors, occupational health professionals, teachers and teaching assistants who are interested in becoming certified to deliver our Mind Health Development workshops, based on our six steps to change your life from within.

For more information or just to drop in and say hello, please visit our website. We'd love to hear from you.

Notes

Introduction

1 Yallom, ID (1985) *The Theory and Practice of Group Therapy*. New York: Basic Books.

Step 1

2 UK Office for National Statistics (2000) *Psychiatric morbidity among adults living in private households in Great Britain*. London: HMSO.
3 Goldberg, D and Huxley, P (1992) *Common mental disorders: a biosocial model*. New York: Routledge.
4 *Diagnostic and Statistical Manual of Mental Disorders text version* (2000). Arlington, VA: American Psychiatric Association.
5 Marano. HE (1999). Depression: beyond serotonin. *Psychology Today*, March 1999.
6 US National Institute of Health Publication Number 00–4501 (1999 reprinted 2000).

7   Schwartz, J (2004). Workplace Stress: Americans' Bugaboo. *New York Times*,
    September 5, p. D2.

8   Murakami, S, Otsuka, K, Kubo, Y, Shinagawa, M, Yamanaka, T, Ohkawa, S
    and Kitaura, Y (2004). Repeated ambulatory monitoring reveals a Monday
    morning surge in blood pressure in a community-dwelling population.
    American Journal of Hypertension, 17 (12) 1179.

9   Chartered Institute of Personnel and Development (2007). *New directions in
    managing employee absence*. London: Chartered Institute of Personnel and
    Development.

10 Health and Safety Executive (2007/2008). *Labour Force Survey*. London:
    HMSO.

11 Deeks, E (2000). Petrol shortage fuels tele-working mini-boom. *People
    Management Magazine* 28 September 2000.

12 UK Office for National Statistics (2010) London: HMSO.

13 WHO Annual Report (2001). *Mental health: new understanding, new hope*.
    Geneva: The World Health Organization.

Step 2

14 Westbrook, D, Kennerley, H and Kirk, J (2008) *An introduction to Cognitive
    Behaviour Therapy*. London: Sage Publications.

15 Burns, D (1980) *Feeling good: the new mood therapy*. New York: Avon
    Paperbacks.

Step 3

16 Rath, T (2007) *Strength Finder 2.0*. New York: Gallup Press.

17 Rath, T and Clifton, D (2004) *How full is your bucket?* New York: Gallup Press.

18 Seligman, MEP and Schulman, P (1986) Explanatory style as a predictor of
    productivity and quitting among life insurance agents. *Journal of Personality
    and Social Psychology* Vol. 50 p. 832.

19 Jones, EE and Harris, VA (1967) The attribution of attitudes. *Journal of
    Experimental Social Psychology* Vol. 3 p. 1.

Step 4

20 Bandler, R and Grinder, J (1975) *The structure of magic*. New York: Science in
    Behaviour Books.

21 Fairweather, AK, Anstey, KJ, Rodgers, B and Butterworth, P (2006) Factors distinguishing suicide attempters from suicide ideators in a community sample: social issues and physical health problems. *Psychological Medicine* Vol. 36 p. 1235.

22 Seligman, MEP (2002) *Authentic Happiness: Using the new positive psychology to realise your potential for lasting fulfilment*, London: Nicholas Brealey Publishing.

Step 5

23 Marmot, M (1994) Work and other factors influencing coronary health and sickness absence. *Work and Stress*, Vol. 8 p. 191.

24 Glasser, W (1998) *Choice Theory*. New York: Harper Perennial.

25 Frankl, V (1946) *Man's search for meaning*. New York: Washington Square Press.

Step 6

26 Norris, RW, Carroll, D, Cochrane, R (1990) The effects of aerobic and anaerobic training on fitness, blood pressure and psychological well-being. *Journal of Psychosomatic Research* Vol. 34 p. 367.

27 Handy, C (1998) *The Hungry Spirit*. London: Arrow Books.

28 Wadell, G and Burton, AK (2006) *Is work good for your well-being? – an evidence review*. London: HMSO.

Index